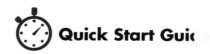
Quick Start Guide

M000114555

The Essential
LOW CARB
HIGH FAT DIET
COOKBOOK

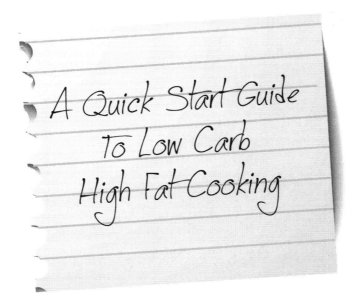

*A Quick Start Guide
To Low Carb
High Fat Cooking*

Over 100 New and Delicious Low Carb High Fat Recipes For Weight Loss

First published in 2015 by Erin Rose Publishing

Text and illustration copyright © 2015 Erin Rose Publishing

Design: Julie Anson

ISBN: 978-0-9933204-2-2

A CIP record for this book is available from the British Library.

DISCLAIMER: This book is for informational purposes only and not intended as a substitute for the medical advice, diagnosis or treatment of a physician or qualified healthcare provider. The reader should consult a physician before undertaking a new health care regime and in all matters relating to his/her health, and particularly with respect to any symptoms that may require diagnosis or medical attention.

While every care has been taken in compiling the recipes for this book we cannot accept responsibility for any problems which arise as a result of preparing one of the recipes. The author and publisher disclaim responsibility for any adverse effects that may arise from the use or application of the recipes in this book. Some of the recipes in this book include nuts and eggs. If you have an egg or nut allergy it's important to avoid these. It is recommended that children, pregnant women, the elderly or anyone who has an immune system disorder avoid eating raw eggs.

CONTENTS

Recipes

Dinner

Desserts & Sweet Treats 97

Condiments 109

INTRODUCTION

'Eat more fat and lose weight? You must be joking!'

Well, we're not but that may have been what you were thinking when you read the title of this book but the low carb high fat diet has gained massive popularity due to its global success.

Fat has been the scapegoat for too long and although it was thought to have been the biggest contributor to weight gain, obesity and type 2 diabetes for decades, all that is radically changing and this revolutionary way of eating is causing such a stir that it can no longer be dismissed as a fad diet. With scientific backing, people worldwide are now discovering for themselves the benefits of low carb high fat eating. They are turning around chronic health problems they thought they were stuck with and losing unwanted weight easily and sustainably. But you don't need to take our word for it - you can try it for yourself!

In this Quick Start Guide we show you how to do it, in simple, easy steps and we provide you with an abundance of delicious, healthy recipes to kick-start weight loss and help you maintain it.

Following on from the success of The Low Carb High Fat Diet we bring you The Essential Low Carb High Fat Diet Cookbook, providing you with another 100 delicious recipes for healthy sustainable weight loss. If you've already read the first book, these recipes will give you added variety and help you to maintain your new way of eating, plus we've included the carbohydrate contents of fruit and vegetables, so that you have all your information in one place. For those of you starting out on the low carb high fat diet – welcome! You've made a great choice.

The LCHF diet doesn't have to be restrictive, lack excitement or even take a long time to prepare. Simple is the way forward. Inside this book you'll find a collection of recipes giving you plenty of ideas for breakfast, lunch and dinner plus snacks and sweet treats.

Are you ready for the low carb high fat challenge? Let's get started!

Getting Started

The sooner you get started the sooner you start losing weight. You can keep it simple to begin with, starting with bacon and eggs for breakfast. Avoid all starchy carbs. Fats should be healthy, natural fats, not margarines and reheated vegetables oils which are dangerous and offer no health benefits. Substitute the carbohydrate portion of your meal for fresh vegetables and add lavish amounts of butter or oil onto them for a satisfying alternative.

As a guide, consume no more than 20g (approx 1oz) of carbs daily to maximise weight loss and to enter ketosis faster. If you are just aiming for the health benefits keep your carbohydrate intake below 50g (2oz) daily.

What Is Ketosis?

Ketosis is a normal metabolic state which occurs when your body doesn't have enough carbohydrates and sugars from your food, causing it to burn fat for energy. This process causes ketones to be released which are excreted in the sweat and urine. Ketostix are available to test if you are in ketosis and therefore burning fat. It's always important to drink plenty of water and especially so to prevent the build up of ketones in the body.

For greater weight loss, avoid fruit as it contains fructose (fruit sugar) but you could introduce this later. Some recipes in this book do contain fruit but they are to be eaten in moderation only. Green leafy vegetables are a great source of fibre, however root vegetables like parsnips and carrots contain more natural sugars. Most people attain significant weight loss without restricting their vegetable intake too much but if your weight loss levels off, it could be that your fruit or vegetable intake is too high.

What Can I Eat?

Foods to AVOID

Below is a list of the food categories detailing which foods to AVOID.

Carbohydrates

- Bread
- Cereals
- Cakes
- Muesli
- Cookies
- Crackers
- Rice cakes
- Oat cakes
- Pasta
- Noodles
- Rice
- Quinoa
- Millet
- Potatoes
- Sweet potatoes

Proteins

- Processed meats such as burgers which aren't 100% beef
- Breaded meat products
- Yogurt unless Greek full-fat (others can contain sugar and little fat)
- Beans and pulses such as kidney beans, butter beans, chickpeas (garbanzo beans), pinto beans, cannellini beans, soy beans and lentils
- Milk, which is less high in fat than other dairy products

Fats

- Corn and canola oil
- Spreads and margarines which are low fat, contain trans fats or contain sugar

Sugars

- Avoid all products containing sugar, syrup, honey, chocolate, sweets and candy. Marinades and readymade sauces like agave syrup, balsamic vinegar, sweet chilli sauces, salad cream, ketchup, barbecue sauce, mustard and any other dressing containing sugar. Always read the labels as sugar is frequently added where you least expect it.

- Avoid dried fruit like apricots, sultanas, raisins and figs.

Drinks

- Steer clear of beer, wine, spirits, cordials, fruit juices, milk, milk shakes, smoothies, fizzy drinks, hot chocolates, oat milk and rice milk.

What Can I Eat?

Foods You CAN Eat

You CAN eat and enjoy the following foods.

Proteins

- Lamb
- Turkey
- Pork
- Eggs
- Beef
- Chicken
- Fish
- Goose
- Venison
- Rabbit

- Fresh fish such as tuna, haddock, cod, anchovies, salmon, trout, sardines, herring and sole.
- Bacon (preferably nitrate & sugar-free)
- Duck
- Shellfish such as prawns, mussels and crab
- Offal
- Tofu
- Nuts and nut butters
- Seeds

Fats

- Butter
- Avocados
- Coconut oil
- Olive oil
- Ghee
- Nut butter

- Full-fat dairy produce; cheeses, Greek yogurt, sour cream, clotted cream, mascarpone, crème fraiche, fresh cream

Fruits

- Apples
- Apricots (fresh)
- Bananas
- Blackberries
- Blueberries

- Cherries
- Grapefruit
- Grapes
- Plums
- Kiwi

Fruits

- Kumquat
- Lemons
- Limes
- Mango
- Melon
- Oranges
- Papaya
- Peaches
- Pears
- Pineapple
- Pomegranate
- Redcurrants
- Strawberries

Don't overdo it with fruit as it can have a high sugar content so eat only occasionally, especially figs, bananas and grapes. Avoid overly ripe fruit which has a higher fructose (fruit sugar) content.

Vegetables

- Root veg; such as parsnips, beet-roots and carrots, in moderation.
- Leeks
- Broccoli
- Cabbage
- Lettuce
- Celery
- Asparagus
- Artichokes
- Aubergine (eggplant)
- Bean sprouts
- Peppers (bell peppers)
- Broad beans
- Cabbage
- Runner beans
- Mushrooms
- Spinach
- Spring onions (scallions)
- Cucumber
- Courgette (zucchini)
- Radish
- Kale
- Cauliflower
- Pak Choi (Bok choy)
- Onions
- Brussels sprouts
- Rocket (arugula)
- Olives
- Watercress

Carbohydrate Contents of Fruit and Vegetables

The following tables of carbohydrate contents of fresh fruits and vegetables are an approximate guide, to help you decide where your carbohydrates come from. Therefore if you can cut back on higher carbohydrate vegetables like carrots and replace them with celery or lettuce, it means you can reduce your carbohydrate intake but still eat plenty of fresh vegetables.

Carbohydrate Content of Vegetables Per 100g

Parsnips	18g	Cabbage	6g
Artichokes	11g	Red peppers (bell pepper)	6g
Beetroot	10g	Cauliflower	5g
Carrots	10g	Green peppers (bell pepper)	4.6g
Swede	9g	Asparagus	3.9g
Brussels sprouts	9g	Tomatoes	3.9g
Kale	9g	Spinach	3.6g
Avocado	9g	Rocket (arugula)	3.6g
Onion	9g	Cucumber	3.6g
Broccoli	7g	Radish	3.4g
Mushrooms	7g	Courgette (zucchini)	3.1g
Green Beans	7g	Celery	3g
Spring Onions (scallions)	7g	Lettuce	2.9g
Pumpkin	6g		
Olives	6g		

Carbohydrate Content of Fruit Per 100g

Figs	28g	Cherries	12g
Bananas	23g	Oranges	12g
Pomegranate	19g	Raspberries	12g
Grapes	17g	Grapefruit	11g
Kumquat	16g	Apricots	11g
Mango	15g	Plums	11g
Kiwi	15g	Nectarines	11g
Pears	15g	Papaya	11g
Redcurrants	14g	Lime	11g
Blueberries	14g	Blackberries	10g
Apples	14g	Lemons	9g
Tangerines	13g	Cantaloupe melon	8g
Pineapple	13g	Strawberries	8g

Carbohydrate Content of Nuts & Seeds Per 100g

Pumpkin seeds	54g	Hazelnuts	17g
Chia seeds	42g	Peanuts	16g
Cashews	30g	Coconuts	15g
Linseeds	29g	Walnuts	14g
Pistachios	28g	Macadamias	14g
Chestnuts	28g	Pine nuts	13g
Sesame seeds	23g	Brazil nuts	12g
Almonds	22g		
Sunflower seeds	20g		

Top Tips To Make It Easy

Remember that fat keeps you feeling satisfied and prevents hunger so don't be afraid of it.

- Plan your meals and snacks in advance to prevent temptation.

- Have plenty of snacks available such as cubes of cheese, rashers of bacon, avocados, olives, a portion of Greek yogurt or some leftovers. Remember your body is using the fat as fuel.

- Eat clean whole healthy foods and quality cuts of meat.

- Replace those carbohydrates with healthy fats, so cook liberally with butter and healthy oils like coconut oil, olive oil and ground nut oils.

- A dollop of cream can be added to your coffee for satisfying fuel boost and you can add a little stevia sweetener if required.

- A spoonful of coconut oil is great for staving off any hunger pangs. Even a cube of butter can stave off hunger which can be especially useful at bedtime.

- Mayonnaise, guacamole or cream cheese can be added to protein and vegetable dishes to boost your fat intake. Replace tortillas and burger baps with iceberg or romaine lettuce leaves.

- You can add extra cream or butter to soups, casseroles and sauces.

- Don't starve yourself. If you are hungry, EAT! You need to keep your metabolism fuelled and starving yourself will slow your metabolism.

- Keep hydrated at all times and water is great for banishing hunger.

- Don't be tempted to increase your fat intake AND still eat starchy carbs. It's a sure way to put on weight.

- For a super-quick snack, beat 2 eggs in a cup with a large knob of butter and microwave it for just under 2 minutes – it's a great snack to keep hunger away.

Recipes

Cooking On A Low Carb High Fat Diet

Cooking and preparing meals on a low carb high fat diet can be quick, easy and packed with flavour. The biggest change may be your portion sizes but where bread, pasta, rice and potatoes have been removed from your meals you can swap them for a portion of vegetables instead. Some of the recipes in this book are for one person, especially the breakfast selection. Not all families have the time to eat together and sometimes everyone wants something different. Other meals are based on four people, so these can either be shared or frozen for another day. This can save you time later when you don't necessarily have a fridge full of ingredients or when you need something quick and easy.

Before you get started, go through your cupboards and check the food labels so that you can eliminate the foods you need to avoid. You could be in for a shock when you discover how much added sugar is in many of your savoury foods. However, by cooking with fresh whole foods, you'll know exactly what's going into your food and you'll have weeded out ingredients which offer little or no nutritional benefit. The aim of this book is to show you how to eat naturally and healthily without highly processed ingredients.

To stop you reaching for unhealthy snacks, prepare for your day by having handy transportable options to stave off hunger pangs. You can check out the recipes and prepare soups and snacks which are easy to store and delicious.

We hope you enjoy finding your favourite recipes. Wishing you great health!

BREAKFAST

Ricotta & Herb Frittata

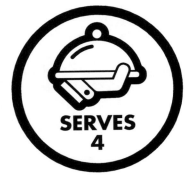

SERVES
4

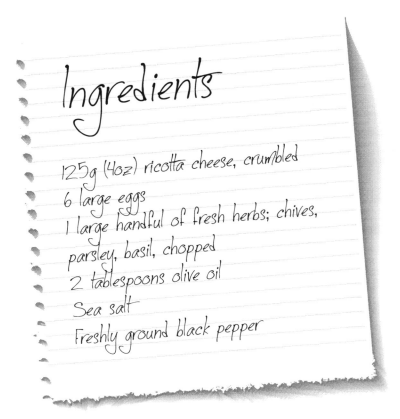

Ingredients

125g (4oz) ricotta cheese, crumbled
6 large eggs
1 large handful of fresh herbs; chives,
parsley, basil, chopped
2 tablespoons olive oil
Sea salt
Freshly ground black pepper

Method

Crack the eggs into a bowl and whisk them. Stir in the fresh herbs and season with salt and pepper. Place the olive oil in a frying pan and pour in the egg mixture and cook them for around 5-6 minutes or until they are set. Sprinkle the ricotta cheese over the eggs and place the pan under a hot grill (broiler) until the top is golden.

Baked Eggs &
Smoked Salmon

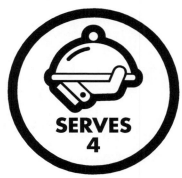

**SERVES
4**

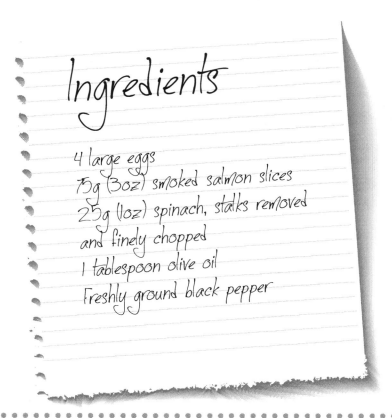

Ingredients

4 large eggs
75g (3oz) smoked salmon slices
25g (1oz) spinach, stalks removed
and finely chopped
1 tablespoon olive oil
Freshly ground black pepper

Method

Heat the olive oil in a pan and add the spinach. Cook for 2 minutes until the spinach has wilted. Line the bases and sides of 4 ramekin dishes with smoked salmon. Divide the spinach between the ramekin dishes then break an egg into each one. Sprinkle with black pepper. Place the ramekins in a preheated oven at 220C/425F for 15 minutes, until the eggs are set.

Feta Cheese & Courgette Omelette

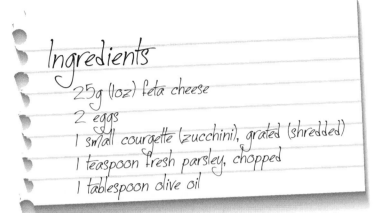

Ingredients

25g (1oz) feta cheese

2 eggs

1 small courgette (zucchini), grated (shredded)

1 teaspoon fresh parsley, chopped

1 tablespoon olive oil

SERVES 1

Method

Place the eggs in a bowl and whisk them. Stir in the cheese and courgette (zucchini). Heat the olive oil in a frying pan. Pour in the egg mixture and cook until it is set. Sprinkle with parsley and serve.

Bacon & Egg Breakfast Peppers

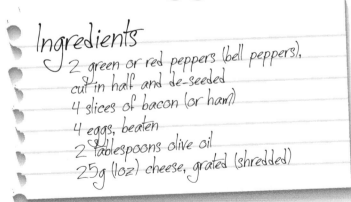

Ingredients

2 green or red peppers (bell peppers), cut in half and de-seeded

4 slices of bacon (or ham)

4 eggs, beaten

2 tablespoons olive oil

25g (1oz) cheese, grated (shredded)

SERVES 4

Method

Place a slice of bacon (or ham) into each pepper half. Pour some of the egg mixture into each of the pepper halves and drizzle with olive oil. Sprinkle the cheese over the peppers. Place the peppers onto a baking sheet and cook in the oven at 190C/375F for around 25 minutes or until the eggs have set.

Spinach Scrambled Eggs

Ingredients

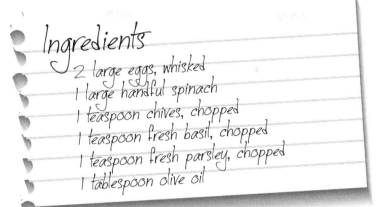

- 2 large eggs, whisked
- 1 large handful spinach
- 1 teaspoon chives, chopped
- 1 teaspoon fresh basil, chopped
- 1 teaspoon fresh parsley, chopped
- 1 tablespoon olive oil

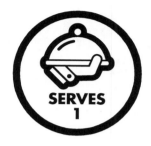

SERVES 1

Method

Heat the oil in a frying pan, add the spinach to the pan and cook for 2 minutes. Combine the herbs with the eggs, pour into the pan with the spinach and stir the mixture until it's lightly scrambled. Season and serve.

Pesto Scrambled Eggs

Ingredients

- 2 large eggs, whisked
- 25g (1oz) cheddar cheese, grated (shredded)
- ½ teaspoon pesto
- 1 tablespoon olive oil
- Sea salt, freshly ground black pepper

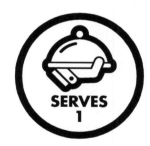

SERVES 1

Method

In a bowl, combine the eggs, cheese and pesto and season with salt and pepper. Heat the oil in a frying pan. Pour in the egg mixture and stir until the eggs are soft but set.

Pancakes, Raspberries & Cream

SERVES 1

Ingredients

125g (4oz) ground almonds (almond flour/ almond meal)

2 eggs, whisked

60mls (2fl oz) water

1 tablespoon olive oil or coconut oil

A few raspberries

1-2 tablespoons of crème fraiche or whipped cream (heavy cream)

Method

Combine all of the ingredients in a bowl except the oil and crème fraiche or cream.
Heat the oil in a frying pan and add some of the pancake batter to the size you require.
Once bubbles begin to appear in the mixture turn it onto the other side. Repeat for the
remaining mixture. Dollop the crème fraiche on top and scatter the raspberries over them.
Enjoy.

Low Carb Breakfast Cereal

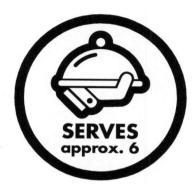

SERVES approx. 6

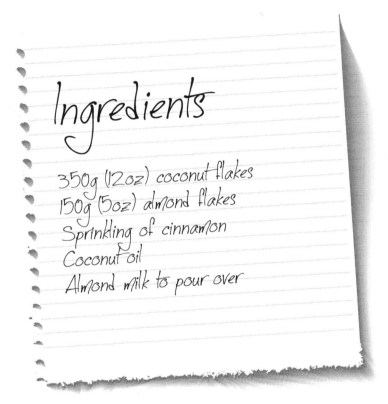

Ingredients

350g (12oz) coconut flakes
150g (5oz) almond flakes
Sprinkling of cinnamon
Coconut oil
Almond milk to pour over

Method

Grease a baking sheet with coconut oil. Spread out the coconut flakes and almond flakes onto the sheet and sprinkle with a little cinnamon. Transfer it to an oven preheated to 180C/360F and bake for 4-5 minutes or until slightly golden. Serve in a bowl and pour over some almond milk and an extra sprinkling of cinnamon if required. You can also swap the almond milk for Greek yogurt or cream.

Lush Mint Smoothie

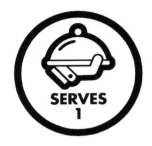

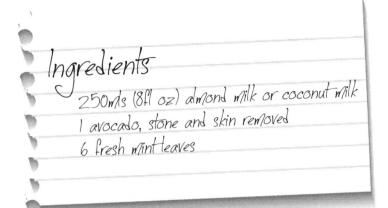

Ingredients

250mls (8fl oz) almond milk or coconut milk
1 avocado, stone and skin removed
6 fresh mint leaves

Method

Place the ingredients into a blender and blitz until smooth. You can add extra almond milk or some water if you like it thinner.

Grapefruit & Spinach Smoothie

SERVES 1

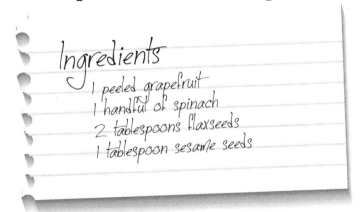

Ingredients

1 peeled grapefruit
1 handful of spinach
2 tablespoons flaxseeds
1 tablespoon sesame seeds

Method

Place all the ingredients into a blender with enough water to cover them and blitz until smooth. If your blender can't grind seeds you can add ground seeds or nuts instead.

Avocado & Ham Omelette

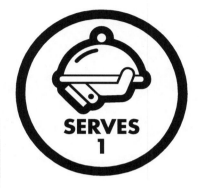

SERVES 1

Ingredients

50g (2oz) cheddar cheese, grated (shredded)
2 eggs, beaten
1 slice of ham, chopped
Flesh of 1/2 avocado, chopped
1 teaspoon crème fraiche
1 tablespoon olive oil
Freshly ground black pepper

Method

Combine the beaten eggs in a bowl with the crème fraiche. Heat the olive oil in a frying pan then pour in the beaten egg mixture. While it begins to set sprinkle on the grated cheese, ham and chopped avocado. Cook until the eggs are completely set and the cheese has melted. Season with black pepper.

Kippers & Mushrooms

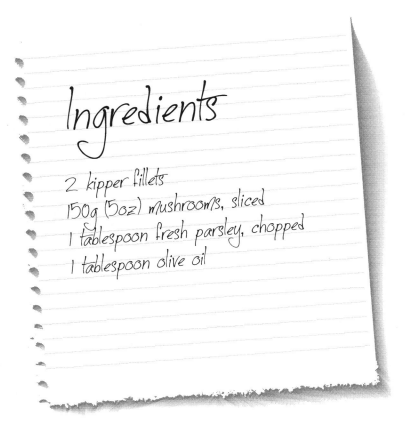

Ingredients

2 kipper fillets
150g (5oz) mushrooms, sliced
1 tablespoon fresh parsley, chopped
1 tablespoon olive oil

SERVES
2

Method

Place the fish under a hot grill (broiler) and cook for around 6 minutes turning halfway through. In the meantime heat the olive oil in a pan, add the chopped mushrooms and cook for 5 minutes until softened. Sprinkle with parsley and serve the fish and mushrooms onto plates.

Crust-Free Quiche

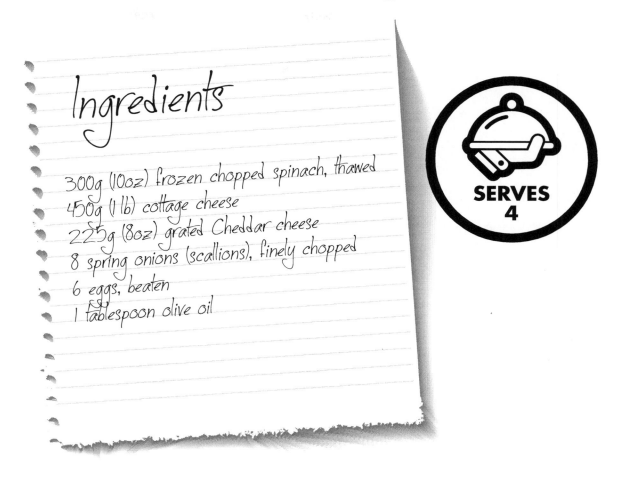

Ingredients

300g (10oz) frozen chopped spinach, thawed
450g (1 lb) cottage cheese
225g (8oz) grated Cheddar cheese
8 spring onions (scallions), finely chopped
6 eggs, beaten
1 tablespoon olive oil

SERVES
4

Method

Lightly grease a quiche dish. Heat a tablespoon of olive oil in a saucepan. Add the spinach and cook until softened. Drain off any excess moisture. Add in the spring onions (scallions), eggs and cheeses and mix well. Pour mixture into prepared quiche dish. Transfer it to an oven preheated to 150C/300F and cook for 50-60 minutes, or until eggs are completely set.

LUNCH

Sesame & Lime Chicken Salad

SERVES 4

Ingredients

4 chicken breasts, cut into strips

1 cucumber, deseeded and chopped

1 handful of coriander (cilantro) leaves, chopped

1 handful of mint leaves, chopped

1 teaspoon ground Szechuan pepper

2 tablespoons sesame oil

4 spring onions (scallions), chopped

Juice of 1 lime

1 bag of mixed lettuce leaves

1 tablespoon olive oil

Method

Heat the olive oil in a pan, add the chicken strips and cook for 8-10 minutes or until the chicken is completely cooked. Remove from the heat and allow it to cool. Place the cucumber and chopped herbs in a bowl with the chicken. Place the sesame oil, pepper, lime juice, spring onions (scallions) in a separate bowl then mix it with the chicken and cucumber. Serve the lettuce onto plates and spoon the chicken mixture on top. Garnish with a little coriander (cilantro).

Herby Grilled
Feta & Asparagus

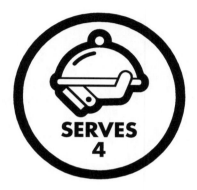

SERVES 4

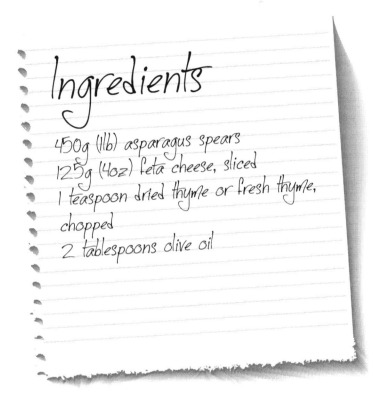

Ingredients

450g (1lb) asparagus spears
125g (4oz) feta cheese, sliced
1 teaspoon dried thyme or fresh thyme,
chopped
2 tablespoons olive oil

Method

Coat the asparagus with a tablespoon of olive oil then place the spears under a hot grill (broiler) and cook for 5 minutes, turning once halfway through. Serve the asparagus onto a plate and place the slices of cheese on top of it. Place the asparagus and feta under the grill (broiler) for 1-2 minutes or until the cheese is beginning to soften. Drizzle a tablespoon of olive oil over the dish and sprinkle with thyme.

Thai Prawn & Coconut Soup

SERVES 4-6

Ingredients

- 450g (1lb) prawns (shrimp), peeled and de-veined
- 4 cloves garlic, crushed
- 5cm (2 inch) chunk of fresh ginger
- 4 teaspoons lemongrass paste or 2 inner stalks, finely chopped
- 1 teaspoon curry powder
- 1/2 teaspoon chilli flakes
- 400mls (14fl oz) vegetable stock (broth)
- 750mls (1 1/4 pints) coconut milk
- 2 tablespoons olive oil
- 1 lime, quartered for garnish
- 1 tablespoon fresh coriander (cilantro)
- Sea salt, freshly ground black pepper

Method

Heat the olive oil in a large saucepan add the ginger, garlic, lemongrass, curry powder and chilli flakes. Cook for around 1 minute. Pour in the stock (broth) and mix well. Bring it to the boil, reduce the heat and simmer gently. Add the prawns and cook for 3 minutes. Pour in the coconut milk and warm it through. Season with salt and pepper. Serve in bowls with a wedge of lime and sprinkle with coriander (cilantro).

Broccoli & Cheese Soup

Ingredients

200g (7oz) cheese, grated (shredded)
1 onion, chopped
1 large head of broccoli, broken into florets
2 tablespoons olive oil
900mls (1½ pints) vegetable stock (broth)
200mls (7fl oz) double cream (heavy cream)
Sea salt
Freshly ground black pepper

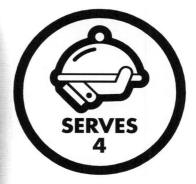

SERVES
4

Method

Heat the olive oil in a saucepan, add the onion and cook for 4 minutes. Add the broccoli and cook for 8 minutes. Stir in the stock (broth) and bring to the boil. Using a food processor or hand blender process until smooth. Stir in the cheese and double cream (heavy cream) and season with salt and pepper.

Turkey & Stilton Soup

Ingredients

350g (12oz) cooked turkey meat

150g (5oz) blue cheese

4 tablespoons butter

1 onion, chopped

1 leek, chopped

1 tablespoon fresh tarragon leaves, chopped

600mls (1 pint) chicken stock (broth)

150mls (5fl oz) double cream (heavy cream)

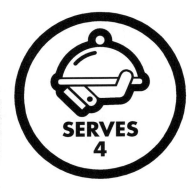

SERVES 4

Method

Heat the butter in a saucepan, add the onion and leek and cook until softened. Add the turkey and stock (broth) to the pan and bring it to the boil. Reduce the heat and simmer for 10 minutes, stirring occasionally. Allow the soup to cool slightly then using a hand blender or food processor blend the soup until it is chunky and smooth. Stir in the blue cheese, double cream (heavy cream) and the chopped tarragon. Heat and stir the soup until warmed through. Serve and enjoy.

Scallop & Leek Soup

Ingredients

150g (5oz) scallops
2 leeks, chopped
1 small courgette (zucchini), chopped
1 large bunch of parsley
2 tablespoons butter
750mls (1¼ pints) chicken stock (broth)
150mls (5fl oz) double cream (heavy cream)
Sea salt
Freshly ground black pepper

SERVES 4

Method

Heat the butter in a frying pan, add the leeks and courgette (zucchini) and cook until softened. Add the chicken stock (broth) and season with salt and pepper. Stir in the parsley and simmer for 10 minutes. Using a hand blender or food processor blitz the soup until smooth. Stir in the cream and bring to the boil. Reduce the heat and add the chopped scallops. Cook them for around 1 minute until the scallops are firm. Serve and enjoy.

Walnut & Cauliflower Soup

SERVES 4

Ingredients

1 head of cauliflower, broken into florets

1 onion, chopped

1 tablespoon butter

4 tablespoons chopped walnuts

600mls (1 pint) vegetable stock (broth)

300mls (½ pint) double cream (heavy cream)
or crème fraiche

½ teaspoon paprika

Sea salt

Freshly ground black pepper

Method

Heat the butter in a saucepan, add the onion and cauliflower and cook for 4 minutes, stirring continuously. Pour in the stock (broth), bring to the boil and cook for 15 minutes until the cauliflower is tender. Add the walnuts, cream and paprika and using a hand blender or food processor blitz the soup until smooth. If using a food processor allow the soup to cool slightly first. Season with salt and pepper. Serve with a sprinkling of chopped nuts and serve.

Barbecue Chicken Wings

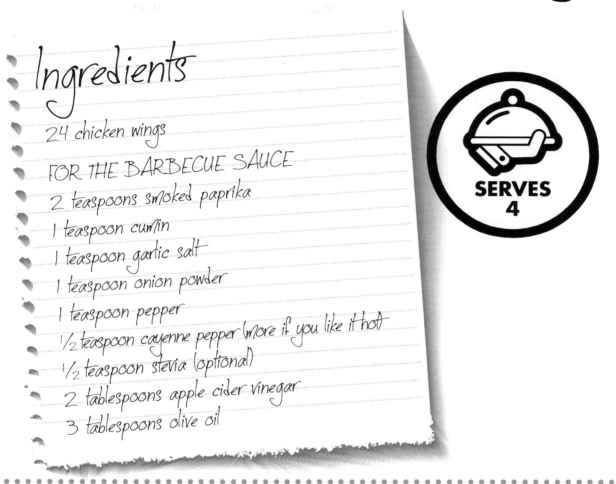

Ingredients

24 chicken wings

FOR THE BARBECUE SAUCE

2 teaspoons smoked paprika

1 teaspoon cumin

1 teaspoon garlic salt

1 teaspoon onion powder

1 teaspoon pepper

1/2 teaspoon cayenne pepper (more if you like it hot)

1/2 teaspoon stevia (optional)

2 tablespoons apple cider vinegar

3 tablespoons olive oil

SERVES
4

Method

In a bowl, combine all the ingredients for the barbecue sauce mixing really well. Preheat the oven to 200C/400F. Coat the chicken wings in the barbecue sauce and then spread them out on a large baking sheet. Place in the oven and bake for around 35 minutes, or until the chicken wings are cooked through and well browned. Serve with dips and salad.

Salmon & Hollandaise Sauce

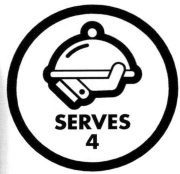

SERVES 4

Ingredients

4 salmon fillets
2 tablespoons chives
2 tablespoons olive oil
Sea salt & freshly ground black pepper

FOR THE HOLLANDAISE SAUCE:
225g (8oz) butter, cut into cubes
3 egg yolks
1 tablespoon water
Juice of 1 lemon
Sea salt & freshly ground black pepper

Method

Combine the olive oil in a bowl with the chives and season with salt and pepper. Coat the salmon fillets in the herb and oil mixture. Place them under a hot grill and cook for around 8 minutes turning once and until cooked thoroughly. To make the hollandaise sauce, place the egg yolks in a heatproof bowl over a saucepan of gently simmering water. Add in the water and season with salt and pepper. Reduce the heat and simmer continuously whisking as the mixture begins to thicken then whisk in the butter a cube at a time until the sauce becomes shiny and thick. Whisk in the lemon juice. Place the grilled salmon onto plates and serve with the hollandaise sauce.

Chilli Chicken Burgers

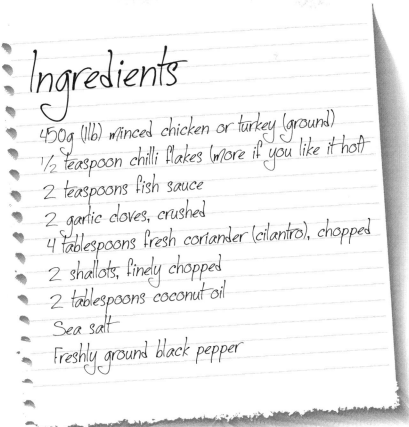

Ingredients

450g (1lb) minced chicken or turkey (ground)

½ teaspoon chilli flakes (more if you like it hot)

2 teaspoons fish sauce

2 garlic cloves, crushed

4 tablespoons fresh coriander (cilantro), chopped

2 shallots, finely chopped

2 tablespoons coconut oil

Sea salt

Freshly ground black pepper

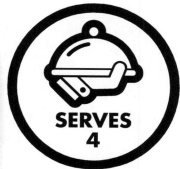

SERVES 4

Method

Place the chicken or turkey in a large bowl and add the coriander (cilantro), fish sauce, garlic, shallots and chilli flakes. Season with salt and pepper. Mix the ingredients together well. Divide the mixture into 4 and form into burger shapes. Heat the coconut oil in a frying pan. Place the burgers in the pan and cook for around 7- 8 minutes on either side until the burgers are cooked through. Serve them in iceberg or romaine lettuce leaves instead of a bread bun. Add a dollop of mayonnaise or guacamole.

Creamy Aubergine & Cheese Bake

Ingredients

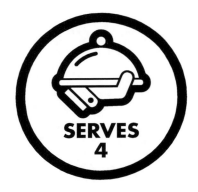

SERVES 4

2 aubergines (eggplants) cut into 2cm slices

150g (5oz) feta cheese, crumbled

150g (5oz) mascarpone cheese

3 eggs

60mls (2fl oz) double cream (heavy cream)

4 tomatoes, sliced

2 tablespoons fresh oregano leaves, chopped

Sea salt

Freshly ground black pepper

Method

Grease and line an ovenproof dish with foil. Place the aubergines (eggplants) in a colander and sprinkle with salt. Allow them to sit for 15 minutes then squeeze off the excess moisture. Line the dish with the aubergine and tomato slices. Place the eggs, feta cheese, mascarpone cheese and double cream (heavy cream) into a bowl and using a hand blender mix until smooth. Pour the creamy mixture over the vegetables and sprinkle with oregano. Season with salt and pepper. Transfer it to the oven and bake at 200C/400F for 35-40 minutes until golden. Serve with a leafy green salad.

Pesto Stuffed Chicken Wrapped in Bacon

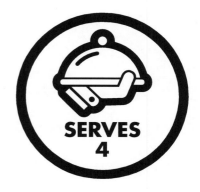

SERVES 4

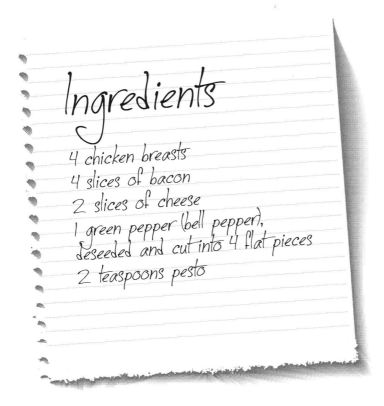

Ingredients

4 chicken breasts
4 slices of bacon
2 slices of cheese
1 green pepper (bell pepper), deseeded and cut into 4 flat pieces
2 teaspoons pesto

Method

Make an incision along the length of the chicken breast and open it up. This will contain the stuffing. Cut or break the cheese and press it fully into the incision. Add the green pepper (bell pepper) on top of the cheese and add a little pesto on top. Fold the chicken breast closed, wrap it in a piece of bacon and secure it with a wooden cocktail stick. Transfer the stuffed chicken breasts to the oven and bake at 180C/360F for around 30 minutes or until the chicken is thoroughly cooked.

Cabbage & Bacon Hash

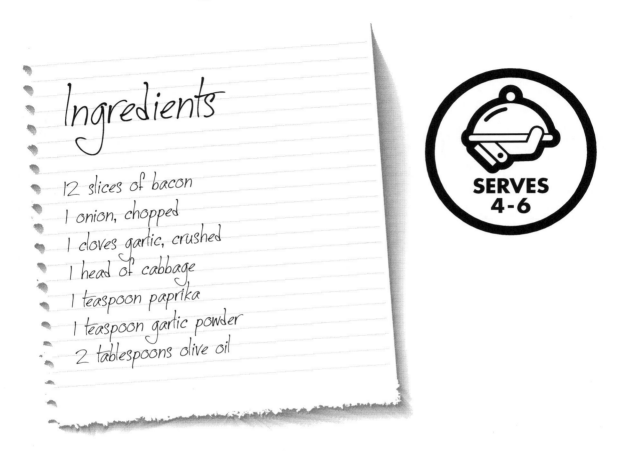

Ingredients

12 slices of bacon
1 onion, chopped
1 cloves garlic, crushed
1 head of cabbage
1 teaspoon paprika
1 teaspoon garlic powder
2 tablespoons olive oil

SERVES 4-6

Method

Place the oil in a large saucepan, add the bacon and cook it for around 8 minutes, until crispy. Add the onion and garlic to the pan and cook for 5 minutes. Add the cabbage to the pan and cook for 10-12 minutes or until softened. Add a little hot water if the you need to add extra moisture to prevent it sticking. Sprinkle in the garlic powder and paprika.

Garlic Dough Balls

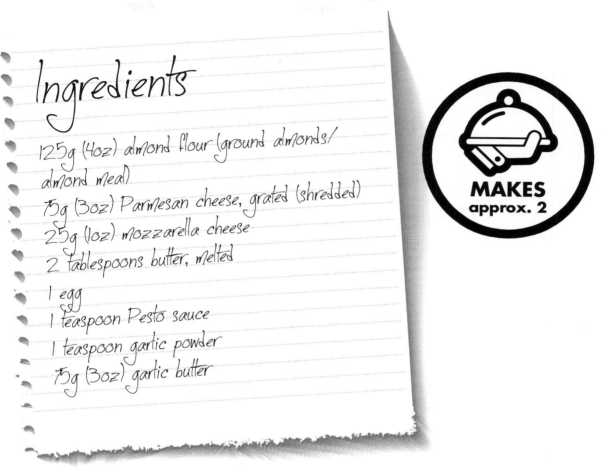

Ingredients

125g (4oz) almond flour (ground almonds/almond meal)

75g (3oz) Parmesan cheese, grated (shredded)

25g (1oz) mozzarella cheese

2 tablespoons butter, melted

1 egg

1 teaspoon Pesto sauce

1 teaspoon garlic powder

75g (3oz) garlic butter

MAKES approx. 2

Method

Place all of the ingredients, apart from the garlic butter, into a bowl and combine them. Grease and line a baking tray. Scoop out a tablespoon of the mixture and roll it into a ball. Repeat it for the remaining mixture. Transfer it to the oven and bake at 180C/360F for around 20 minutes, or until golden. Spread some garlic butter onto each dough ball. Enjoy warm.

Chicken & Avocado Burgers

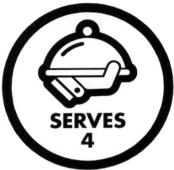

SERVES 4

Ingredients

450g (1lb) minced (ground) chicken or turkey

50g (2oz) ground almonds (almond meal/almond flour)

2 cloves of garlic, crushed

1 large ripe avocado, skin and stone removed, cut into small chunks

Sea salt

Freshly ground black pepper

Method

Place all of the ingredients into a bowl and combine them well. Scoop out the mixture and shape it into patties. Transfer the burgers to a hot grill (broiler) and cook for around 10 minutes, turning once half way through. Serve with guacamole and roast vegetables.

Mozzarella Breadsticks

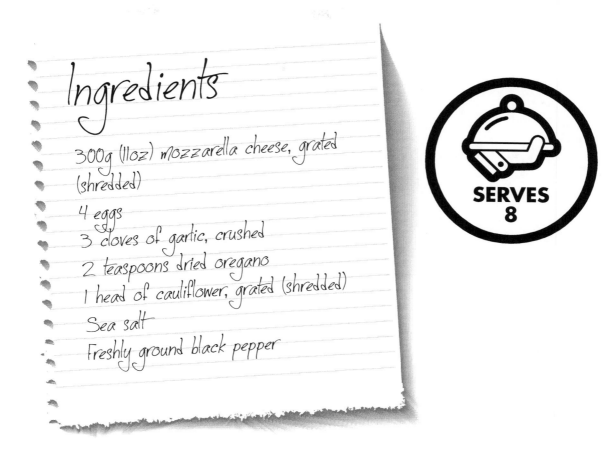

Ingredients

300g (11oz) mozzarella cheese, grated (shredded)

4 eggs

3 cloves of garlic, crushed

2 teaspoons dried oregano

1 head of cauliflower, grated (shredded)

Sea salt

Freshly ground black pepper

SERVES 8

Method

Steam the cauliflower for 5 minutes or until tender and allow it to cool. Place the cauliflower in a bowl and combine it with the eggs, two thirds of the cheese, oregano and garlic. Season with salt and pepper. Grease 2 baking sheets. Divide the mixture in half and place it on the baking sheet and press it into a flat rectangular shape. Transfer the baking sheets to the oven and bake at 220C/440F for 20-25 minutes or until slightly golden. Remove them from the oven and sprinkle them with the remaining mozzarella cheese. Return them to the oven for 4-5 minutes or until the cheese has melted. Cut the breads into sticks or slices of a size to your liking.

Halloumi & Asparagus Salad

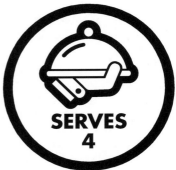

SERVES 4

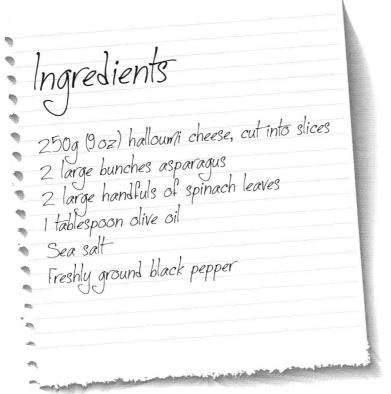

Ingredients

250g (9oz) halloumi cheese, cut into slices
2 large bunches asparagus
2 large handfuls of spinach leaves
1 tablespoon olive oil
Sea salt
Freshly ground black pepper

Method

Heat the olive oil in a frying pan and cook the asparagus for 4 minutes or until tender. Remove, set aside and keep warm. Place the halloumi in the frying pan and cook for 2 minutes on each side until golden. Serve the spinach leaves onto plates and add the asparagus and halloumi slices. Season with salt and pepper. Drizzle with extra olive oil.

Aubergine & Feta Salad

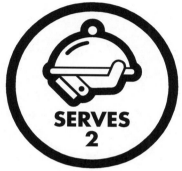

SERVES 2

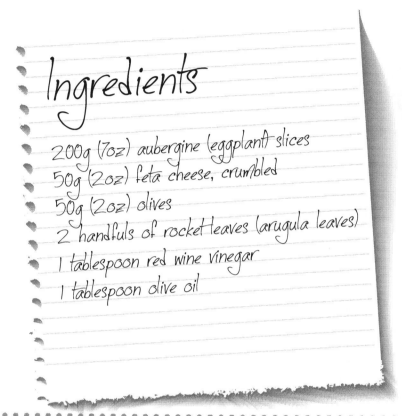

Ingredients

200g (7oz) aubergine (eggplant) slices

50g (2oz) feta cheese, crumbled

50g (2oz) olives

2 handfuls of rocket leaves (arugula leaves)

1 tablespoon red wine vinegar

1 tablespoon olive oil

Method

Heat a tablespoon of olive oil in griddle pan or barbecue and add the aubergine (eggplant). Cook for around 3-4 minutes until tender. Place it in a bowl and allow it to cool slightly. Add the feta cheese, olives and rocket (arugula). In a separate bowl mix together the tablespoon of olive oil, vinegar then pour it onto the aubergine salad. Serve.

Mini Cauliflower Pizza Bases

SERVES 4-6

Ingredients

- 450g (1 lb) mozzarella cheese, grated (shredded)
- 2 eggs
- 1 head of cauliflower, grated (shredded)
- 1 teaspoon dried oregano
- 1 teaspoon dried basil
- 1 teaspoon garlic powder
- 1 tomato, sliced
- Handful of fresh basil leaves, chopped
- 200mls (7fl oz) passata/tomato sauce

Method

Steam the grated (shredded) cauliflower for 5 minutes then allow it to cool. Place the cooked cauliflower in a bowl and add the eggs, half the cheese, dried herbs and garlic and mix everything together really well. Grease two baking sheets. Divide the mixture into 12 and roll it into balls. Place them on a baking sheet and press them down until flat and round mini pizza bases. Transfer them to the oven and bake at 220C/440F for 12 minutes until lightly golden.

Top each pizza base with a little passata, mozzarella and tomato and basil. Place the pizzas under a grill (broiler) and cook for 4-5 minutes or until the cheese has melted. Enjoy.

Mackerel Kebabs

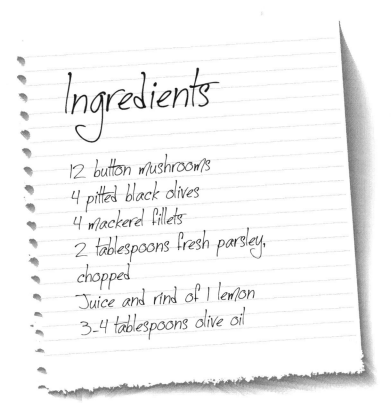

Ingredients

12 button mushrooms
4 pitted black olives
4 mackerel fillets
2 tablespoons fresh parsley, chopped
Juice and rind of 1 lemon
3-4 tablespoons olive oil

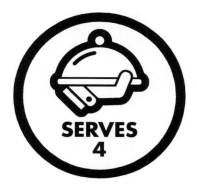

SERVES
4

Method

Cut the fish into chunks and place them in a bowl. Squeeze in the lemon juice and add the rind, olive oil and parsley and coat the fish chunks thoroughly. Add the mushrooms and coat them in the dressing too. Thread the fish chunks and mushrooms onto skewers and add an olive at the end. Place the kebabs under a hot grill (broiler) and cook for 4-5 minutes turning occasionally. Serve the kebabs and drizzle them with the remaining dressing.

Ham & Cream Cheese
Bread-Free Sandwich

Ingredients
3 slices of ham
2 tablespoons cream cheese
1 cucumber, peeled, seeds removed and
halved lengthways
1 tablespoon chives, chopped

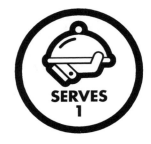

SERVES
1

Method

Spread each half of cucumber with cream cheese and sprinkle the chopped chives onto the cheese. Layer the ham on one half of the cucumber and place the other half on top, using it as a lid like you would a bread sandwich. Cut in half widthways. Eat straight away.

Turkey & Cheddar
Bread-Free Sandwich

Ingredients
2 slices of turkey
2 thick slices cheddar cheese
1 red pepper (bell pepper),
cut into quarters and de-seeded

SERVES
1

Method

Flatten each piece of pepper (bell pepper) slightly. Lay 2 pieces of pepper flat, add a layer of turkey and a layer of cheese. Use the 2 remaining pieces of pepper as a lid and cover the turkey and cheese as you would a bread sandwich.

Pine Nut & Avocado Salad

SERVES 2

Ingredients

4 tablespoons pine nuts, roughly chopped
2 avocados, peeled, stone removed and thickly sliced
2 baby Cos lettuces, trimmed
1 tablespoon lemon juice
1 teaspoon olive oil
2 tablespoons olive oil
3 teaspoons white wine vinegar
Sea salt
Freshly ground black pepper

Method

Heat 1 teaspoon of olive oil in a frying pan, add the pine nuts and cook until slightly golden. Coat the avocados with lemon juice. Place the lettuce leaves on a serving plate and scatter the avocado on top. Combine the remaining olive oil, vinegar and salt and pepper in a bowl and mix well. Drizzle the oil over salad and sprinkle over the pine nuts.

Broccoli & Egg Salad

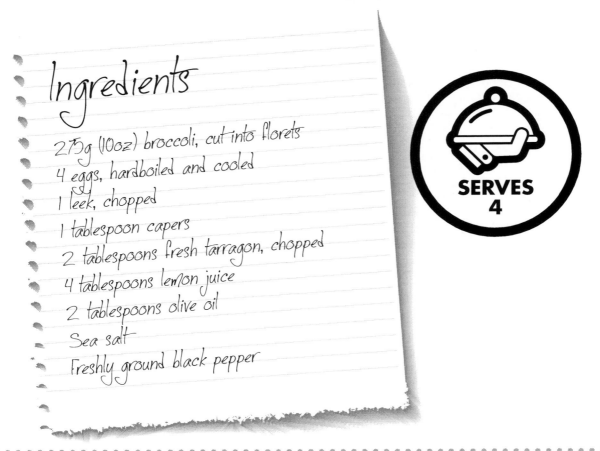

Ingredients

275g (10oz) broccoli, cut into florets
4 eggs, hardboiled and cooled
1 leek, chopped
1 tablespoon capers
2 tablespoons fresh tarragon, chopped
4 tablespoons lemon juice
2 tablespoons olive oil
Sea salt
Freshly ground black pepper

SERVES 4

Method

Place the broccoli into a steamer and cook for 3 minutes. Add the leek and cook for a further 2 minutes. Place the lemon juice, capers, oil and tarragon into a bowl and season with salt and pepper. Remove the shells from the hard-boiled eggs and chop them roughly. Place the broccoli and leeks into the bowl and toss them in the dressing. Serve the salad and sprinkle with the chopped eggs.

Chicken & Parma Ham Rolls

Ingredients

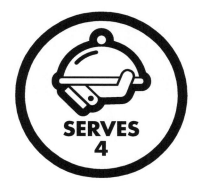

SERVES 4

450g (1lb) blue cheese
300g (11oz) frozen spinach, drained
8 slices Parma ham
4 shallots, finely chopped
4 large chicken breasts, skinless
4 tablespoons butter
1 egg, whisked
1 tablespoon fresh oregano, chopped
1 tablespoon fresh chives, chopped

Method

Heat 2 tablespoons of butter in a frying pan, add the shallots and cook until softened. Allow them to cool. Place the spinach in a bowl with the blue cheese, cooked shallots, egg and herbs and combine well. Cut each chicken breast in half and flatten it out, pounding if necessary. Place some of the cheese mixture into the middle of each chicken breast and then roll them up. Wrap a slice of ham around the chicken roll and secure it with a wooden cocktail stick. Place the chicken rolls on a baking sheet and coat them with the remaining butter. Transfer them to an oven, preheated to 180C/360F and cook them until slightly golden and cooked through.

Almond Stuffed Avocados

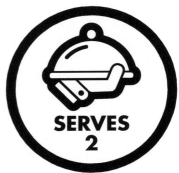

SERVES 2

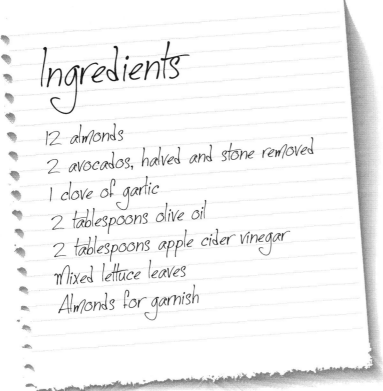

Ingredients

12 almonds
2 avocados, halved and stone removed
1 clove of garlic
2 tablespoons olive oil
2 tablespoons apple cider vinegar
Mixed lettuce leaves
Almonds for garnish

Method

Place the almonds, garlic, oil and vinegar into a food processor and blitz until smooth. Spoon the mixture into the hollows of the avocados. Garnish with an almond on top and serve onto a bed of lettuce.

Lemon Chicken Skewers

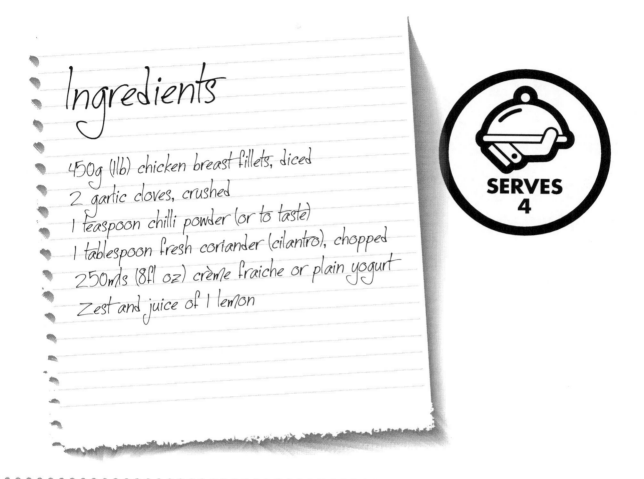

Ingredients

450g (1lb) chicken breast fillets, diced
2 garlic cloves, crushed
1 teaspoon chilli powder (or to taste)
1 tablespoon fresh coriander (cilantro), chopped
250mls (8fl oz) crème fraiche or plain yogurt
Zest and juice of 1 lemon

SERVES 4

Method

Place the crème fraiche/yogurt into a bowl and stir in the garlic, lemon zest and juice, chilli powder and coriander (cilantro). Add in the chicken chunks and mix well. Allow the chicken to marinate for at least 1 hour or overnight if you can. Thread the chicken onto skewers. Place them under a hot grill (broiler) or barbecue and cook for around 4 minutes on each side until the chicken is thoroughly cooked. Serve with a generous dollop of lemon and chilli mayonnaise (see recipe).

Spinach, Cheese & Walnut Salad

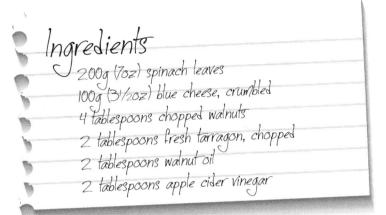

Ingredients
- 200g (7oz) spinach leaves
- 100g (3½oz) blue cheese, crumbled
- 4 tablespoons chopped walnuts
- 2 tablespoons fresh tarragon, chopped
- 2 tablespoons walnut oil
- 2 tablespoons apple cider vinegar

SERVES 4

Method

Mix the vinegar, walnut oil, spinach and tarragon in a bowl and coat the leaves well. Add the walnuts and cheese to the salad and serve.

Radish & Fennel Salad

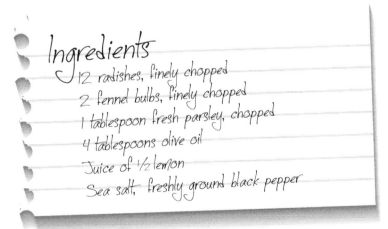

Ingredients
- 12 radishes, finely chopped
- 2 fennel bulbs, finely chopped
- 1 tablespoon fresh parsley, chopped
- 4 tablespoons olive oil
- Juice of ½ lemon
- Sea salt, freshly ground black pepper

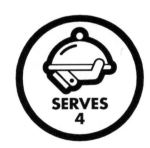

SERVES 4

Method

Place the chopped radishes and fennel into a bowl. Add the lemon juice, olive oil and parsley and stir well. Season with salt and pepper and serve.

Chicory & Blue Cheese Boats

Ingredients

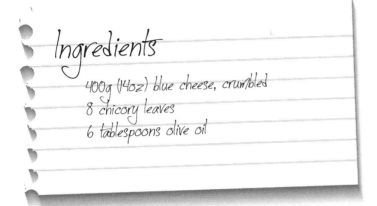

400g (14oz) blue cheese, crumbled
8 chicory leaves
6 tablespoons olive oil

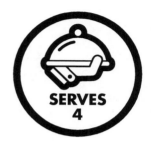

SERVES
4

Method

Place the chicory leaves onto a large baking sheet. Scatter the cheese inside the leaves and drizzle them with olive oil. Place them under a hot grill (broiler) for around 5 minutes, or until the cheese has melted and the chicory slightly golden. Serve and eat immediately.

Roast Courgettes (Zucchinis)

Ingredients

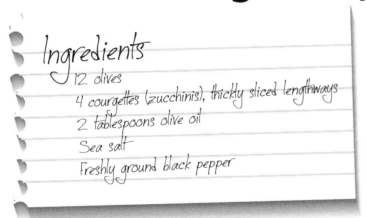

12 olives
4 courgettes (zucchinis), thickly sliced lengthways
2 tablespoons olive oil
Sea salt
Freshly ground black pepper

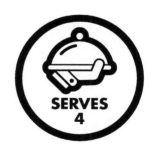

SERVES
4

Method

Place the courgette (zucchini) slices in an ovenproof dish and scatter over the olives. Drizzle with olive oil and season with salt and pepper. Transfer them to the oven and bake at 200C/400F for 15 minutes, turning halfway through.

Crab Pate

Ingredients

125g (4oz) butter
150g (5oz) cream cheese
300g (11oz) crab meat
2 tablespoons chives
1 tablespoon capers
1 shallot, chopped
2 tablespoons lemon juice
Sea salt
Freshly ground black pepper

SERVES 4

Method

Place the butter, shallot, cream cheese and lemon juice into a blender and process lightly under well combined. Transfer them mixture to a bowl and stir in the crab meat, capers and chives. Season with salt and pepper. Chill and serve alongside raw vegetable crudities.

Herby Baked Ricotta & Green Salad

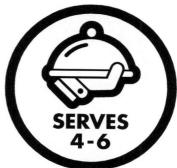

SERVES 4-6

Ingredients

- 900g (2lb) ricotta cheese
- 3 eggs, whisked
- 2 tablespoons fresh chives or parsley
- 1 bag of fresh salad leaves
- 1/2 teaspoon paprika
- Sea salt
- Freshly ground black pepper

Method

Grease a loaf tin with a little oil. Place the ricotta cheese into a bowl and beat to make it soften. Pour in the eggs and combine with the cheese then add in the herbs and paprika and mix well. Season with salt and pepper. Scoop the mixture into the loaf tin and cook in the oven at 180C/360F for 30-35 minutes or until firm. Allow the baked ricotta to cool before removing it from the tin. Slice it and serve with the salad leaves.

Hake & Lime Butter

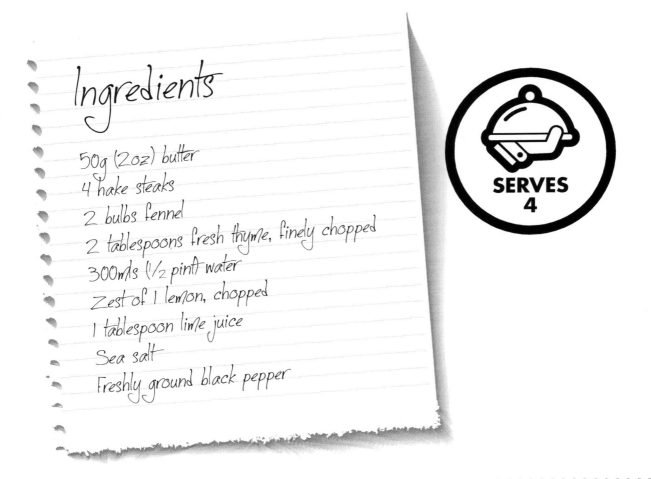

Ingredients

50g (2oz) butter
4 hake steaks
2 bulbs fennel
2 tablespoons fresh thyme, finely chopped
300mls (½ pint) water
Zest of 1 lemon, chopped
1 tablespoon lime juice
Sea salt
Freshly ground black pepper

SERVES 4

Method

Place the fennel, thyme, lemon zest and water into an ovenproof dish. Place the butter in a small bowl and mix in the lime juice. Coat the fish with the lime butter then place the fish on top of the fennel. Season with salt and pepper. Cover the dish with foil and bake in the oven at 200C/400F for 35 minutes, turning the fish over halfway through. Remove the foil and cook for another 5 minutes. Serve with green salad.

Fried Avocado Wedges & Lime Dip

Ingredients

2 large avocados, skin and stone removed and cut into wedges

200g (7oz) ground almonds (almond meal)

1 egg, beaten

1 tablespoon olive oil

FOR THE DIP:

100g (3½oz) Greek yogurt

1 tablespoon fresh coriander (cilantro), chopped

Juice of ½ lime

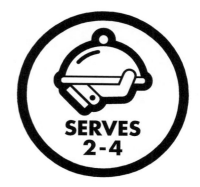

SERVES
2-4

Method

Place the beaten egg in a bowl and place the ground almonds in another bowl. Grease a baking sheet with olive oil. Dip the avocado wedges in the egg then dredge them in the ground almonds. Lay the wedges out on the baking sheet. Transfer them to the oven and bake at 220C/440F for 10-12 minutes until golden. Combine the ingredients for the dip in a bowl and mix well. Serve the avocado wedges hot alongside the dip.

Turkey Lettuce Wrap

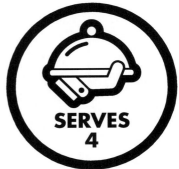

SERVES 4

Ingredients

4 leaves iceberg lettuce
4 slices roast turkey
½ cucumber, sliced
2 tablespoons mayonnaise
Sprinkling of paprika

Method

Top a lettuce leaf with a slice of turkey, cucumber, mayo and paprika, then, as if it were a sandwich, wrap it up with another piece of lettuce. Repeat with the remaining ingredients.

Alternatively try this with avocados, smoked salmon, prawns, leftover chicken, cheese and herbs.

DINNER

Low Carb Lasagne

Ingredients

- 450g (1lb) minced beef (ground beef)
- 275g (10oz) cream cheese; ricotta or mascarpone
- 150g (5oz) mozzarella cheese, grated (shredded)
- 3 tablespoons Parmesan cheese
- 3 garlic cloves, crushed
- 1 onion, finely chopped
- 1 egg
- 1 handful of spinach, washed and finely chopped
- 400g (14oz) passata
- 1 tablespoon olive oil
- Sea salt
- Freshly ground black pepper

SERVES 6-8

Method

Heat the olive oil in a large saucepan, add the beef and brown it. Add in the garlic, passata and season with salt and pepper. In the meantime place the cream cheese in a bowl and beat it to soften it. Add the egg and combine it with the cheese. Stir in the spinach to the cheese mixture. Spoon HALF the meat mixture into a casserole dish and spread the cheese/spinach mixture on top. Add another layer of meat and sprinkle over half the mozzarella, followed by another layer of meat. Top it off with mozzarella and a sprinkling of parmesan. Transfer it to a pre-heated oven and cook for 30 minutes until golden and the cheese is bubbling. Serve with a heap of green salad leaves.

Lemon & Bacon Stuffed Pork

SERVES 4

Ingredients

450g (1lb) thick pork fillets
100g (3½oz) bacon, chopped
2 tablespoons ground almonds
1 onion, finely chopped
1 clove garlic, crushed
1 tablespoon fresh oregano, chopped
1 tablespoon olive oil
1 tablespoon butter
Grated zest of 2 lemons
200mls (7fl oz) chicken stock (broth)

Method

Cut an incision in each piece of pork. Place the almonds, lemon zest, butter, bacon, garlic and oregano in a bowl and combine the mixture. Spoon the stuffing into the pork fillets. Heat the olive oil in a pan, add the onion and cook it for 5 minutes until softened. Add the pork and brown it all over. Pour in the stock (broth) and cook until the pork is cooked through. Serve with steamed or roast vegetables.

Tuna Steaks & Herb Dressing

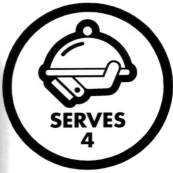

SERVES 4

Ingredients

4 tuna steaks
1 tablespoon fresh parsley
Juice and grated (shredded) rind of 1 lemon
2 tablespoons olive oil

FOR THE DRESSING:
25g (1oz) pitted green olives
1 tablespoon fresh parsley, chopped
1 tablespoon fresh chives, chopped
1 tablespoon fresh coriander (cilantro), chopped
2 tablespoons olive oil
2 tablespoons lemon juice

Method

Combine the juice and rind of the lemon, 1 tablespoon of parsley and 2 tablespoons of olive oil in a bowl and coat the tuna steaks with the mixture. Heat a frying pan or griddle pan on a high heat, add the tuna steaks and cook them for 2-3 minutes on either side or less if you prefer them rare. In the meantime combine the ingredients for the dressing in a bowl and mix well. Serve the tuna steaks with a spoonful of the dressing on the side. Goes beautifully with a mixed salad.

Smoked Fish & Vegetable Gratin

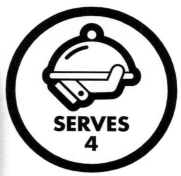

SERVES 4

Ingredients

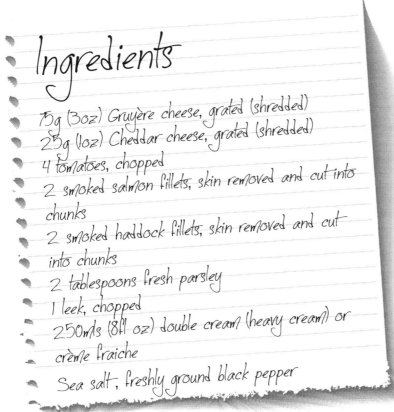

- 75g (3oz) Gruyère cheese, grated (shredded)
- 25g (1oz) Cheddar cheese, grated (shredded)
- 4 tomatoes, chopped
- 2 smoked salmon fillets, skin removed and cut into chunks
- 2 smoked haddock fillets, skin removed and cut into chunks
- 2 tablespoons fresh parsley
- 1 leek, chopped
- 250mls (8fl oz) double cream (heavy cream) or crème fraiche
- Sea salt, freshly ground black pepper

Method

Place the chopped leeks and tomatoes in the bottom of a casserole dish. Add a layer of fish chunks on top of the vegetables and season with salt and pepper. Sprinkle the cheeses and parsley on top then pour over the cream. Transfer it to the oven and bake at 220C/425F for 20-25 minutes or until the cheese is bubbling and the fish is thoroughly cooked.

Almond Chicken Curry

Ingredients

100g (3½ oz) ground almonds (almond flour/
almond meal)
4 chicken breasts, diced
2 teaspoon garam masala
2 onions, peeled and quartered
2 tsp finely grated fresh ginger
2 teaspoons ground cumin
1 teaspoon ground coriander (cilantro)
1 teaspoon ground turmeric
½ teaspoon ground cinnamon
250mls (8fl oz) water
120mls (4fl oz) double cream (heavy cream)
1 tablespoon coconut oil
Toasted almond flakes to garnish

**SERVES
4**

Method

Combine the ground almonds (almond meal) and water in medium bowl and set aside. Heat the coconut oil in a large saucepan. Add the onion and ginger and cook for 5 minutes. Add the cumin, coriander (cilantro), turmeric, cinnamon and cook for 1 minute. Add the chicken and the ground almond mixture. Bring it to the boil, reduce the heat and simmer for 25-30 minutes until the chicken is thoroughly cooked and the sauce has thickened. Add the cream and garam masala and cook for a further 10 minutes. Remove from heat. Sprinkle chicken curry with flaked almonds and serve with cauliflower rice.

Prawn & Seafood Coconut Stew

Ingredients

450g (1lb) white fish fillets, cut into chunks
450g (1lb) large prawns (shrimps), peeled but tails intact
1 small handful fresh coriander (cilantro), chopped
4cm (2 inch) chunk of ginger, peeled, finely chopped
4 garlic cloves, crushed
2 red chillies, thinly sliced
1 onion, chopped
1 green pepper (bell pepper), chopped
1 red pepper (bell pepper), chopped
200mls (7fl oz) coconut milk
120mls (4fl oz) chicken stock (broth)
1 tablespoon olive oil
1 lime, juiced
Fresh coriander (cilantro) leaves, to garnish

SERVES
4-6

Method

Heat the oil in a saucepan over medium-low heat. Cook the onion for 3 minutes or until soft. Stir in the red and green peppers (bell peppers), ginger, garlic and chilli and cook for 3 minutes. Stir in coconut milk and stock (broth). Bring to the boil. Reduce heat to low. Add the fish and simmer for 2-3 minutes. Add the prawns and simmer for 3-4 minutes or until cooked. Stir in the chopped coriander (cilantro) and lime juice. Garnish with coriander leaves.

Thai Beef

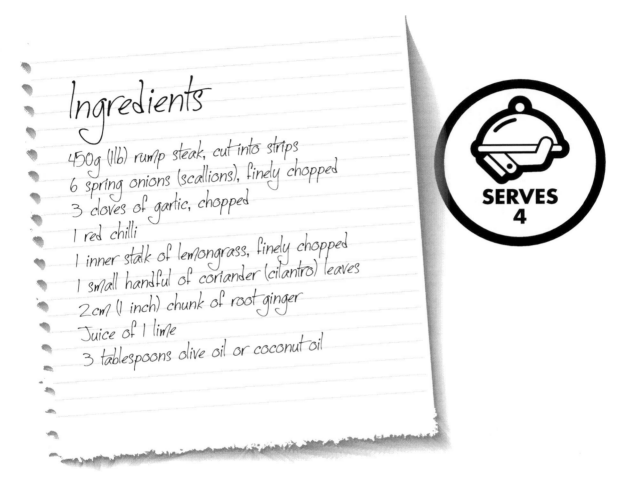

Ingredients

450g (1lb) rump steak, cut into strips
6 spring onions (scallions), finely chopped
3 cloves of garlic, chopped
1 red chilli
1 inner stalk of lemongrass, finely chopped
1 small handful of coriander (cilantro) leaves
2cm (1 inch) chunk of root ginger
Juice of 1 lime
3 tablespoons olive oil or coconut oil

SERVES 4

Method

Place the lemongrass, chilli, garlic, ginger and 2 tablespoons of oil into a blender and blitz until smooth. Place the steak in a bowl and add the lemongrass mixture, coating it well to coat the beef. Marinate for 30 minutes or longer if you can. Heat the remaining oil in a frying pan or wok and add the beef, lime juice. Cook for 5-6 minutes or until cooked through. Sprinkle with spring onions (scallions) and coriander (cilantro) and serve.

Celeriac Mash

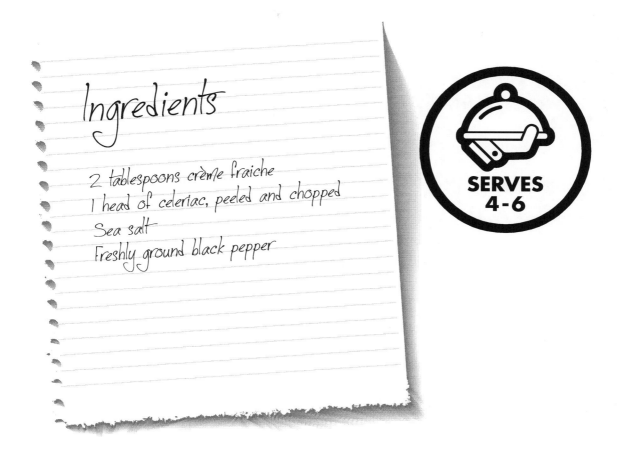

Ingredients

2 tablespoons crème fraiche
1 head of celeriac, peeled and chopped
Sea salt
Freshly ground black pepper

SERVES 4-6

Method

Place the celeriac in a saucepan and boil it for 20 minutes, then drain off the water. Mash the celeriac until smooth then stir in the crème fraiche. Season with salt and pepper. Serve as a low carb alternative to potato mash as an accompaniment to meat dishes.

Greek Lamb Skewers & Feta Salad

Ingredients

450g (1lb) lamb steaks, cut into chunks
2 tablespoons fresh oregano, chopped
1 tablespoon fresh rosemary leaves, chopped
1 clove of garlic, crushed (optional)
Juice and rind of 1 lemon
2 tablespoons olive oil

FOR THE SALAD:
225g (8oz) feta cheese
1 onion, finely chopped
1 cucumber, finely chopped
3 tablespoons fresh parsley, chopped
2 tablespoons olive oil

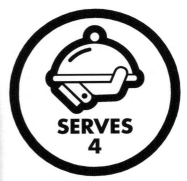

SERVES
4

Method

Place the lemon juice, rind, oregano, rosemary, olive oil and garlic (if using) into a bowl, add the lamb chunks and coat them well. Thread the lamb onto skewers and place them under a hot grill (broiler) for around 8 minutes, turning occasionally until cooked through. In the meantime, place the cucumber, feta, parsley, onion and olive oil in a bowl and combine the ingredients. Serve the salad onto plates and place the lamb kebabs alongside.

Baked Scallops

Ingredients

600g (1lb 5oz) shelled scallops, roughly chopped

25g (1oz) cheddar cheese, grated (shredded)

2 garlic cloves, crushed

2 tablespoons fresh parsley, chopped (plus extra for garnish)

1 onion, finely chopped

Pinch of ground nutmeg

Pinch of ground cloves

2 tablespoons olive oil

SERVES 4

Method

Place the chopped scallops, garlic, onion, parsley, cloves and nutmeg into a bowl and mix well. Using 4 clean scallop shells, or 4 serving dishes, spoon the scallop mixture into them. Pour over ½ tablespoon of olive oil into each shell/dish. Sprinkle with cheese and parsley. Transfer them to the oven and bake at 200C/400F for around 20 minutes or until golden.

Bacon Crusted Meatloaf

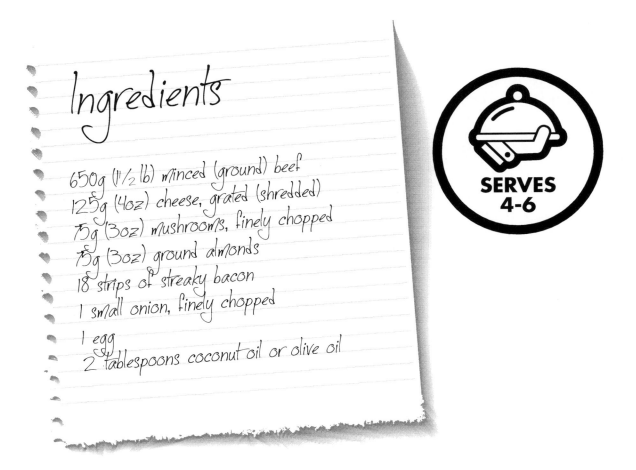

Ingredients

650g (1½ lb) minced (ground) beef
125g (4oz) cheese, grated (shredded)
75g (3oz) mushrooms, finely chopped
75g (3oz) ground almonds
18 strips of streaky bacon
1 small onion, finely chopped
1 egg
2 tablespoons coconut oil or olive oil

SERVES 4-6

Method

Place the meat, mushrooms, onion, almonds, cheese and egg in a food processor and combine them. Line a loaf tin with cling film and press the mixture into the tin and cover it with film too. This is to get the shape of the loaf first. Remove the meat loaf from the tin and place it on a wire rack on a baking tray. Remove the plastic film. Lay the bacon rashers over the meat loaf, completely covering it and tucking the edges of the bacon underneath the loaf. Bake the meat loaf in an oven pre-heated to 180C/360F for 1 hour, or until the meat is completely cooked.

Lemon Sole & Herb Butter

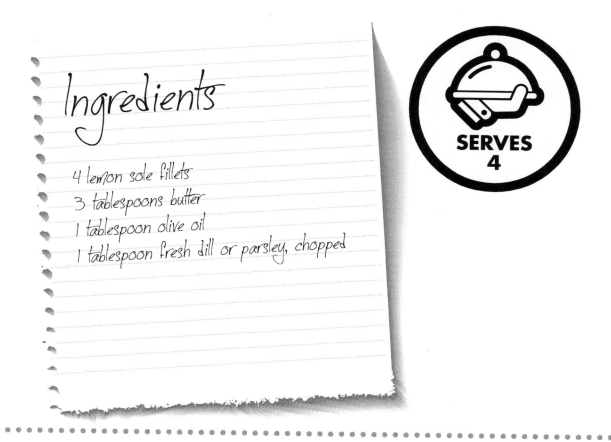

SERVES 4

Ingredients

- 4 lemon sole fillets
- 3 tablespoons butter
- 1 tablespoon olive oil
- 1 tablespoon fresh dill or parsley, chopped

Method

Grease and ovenproof dish with olive oil and lay the fish in it. In a bowl, combine the butter and herbs then spoon the mixture over the fish. Transfer it to the oven and bake at 180C/360F for 20 minutes or until cooked through.

Jerk Chicken Wings & Salsa

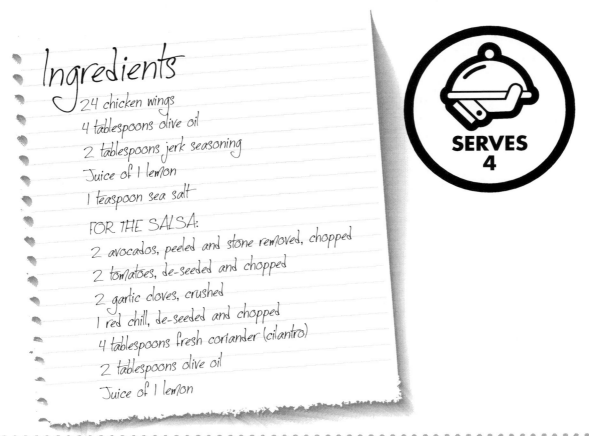

Ingredients

24 chicken wings

4 tablespoons olive oil

2 tablespoons jerk seasoning

Juice of 1 lemon

1 teaspoon sea salt

FOR THE SALSA:

2 avocados, peeled and stone removed, chopped

2 tomatoes, de-seeded and chopped

2 garlic cloves, crushed

1 red chill, de-seeded and chopped

4 tablespoons fresh coriander (cilantro)

2 tablespoons olive oil

Juice of 1 lemon

SERVES 4

Method

Place the chicken wings into a bowl and sprinkle them with jerk seasoning. Stir in the olive oil, lemon juice and salt and coat them really well in the mixture. Allow to marinate for 1 hour or overnight if you can. In the meantime place all of the ingredients for the salsa into a bowl and combine them. Place the chicken wings under a hot grill (boiler) and cook them for 10-12 minutes, turning once halfway through. Serve the chicken wings with the salsa on the side.

Lamb & Spinach Curry

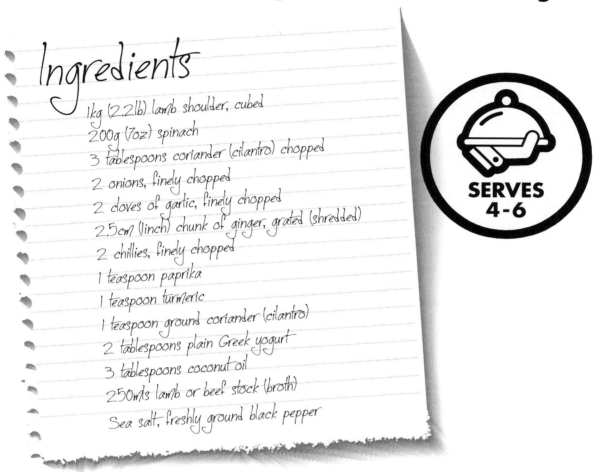

Ingredients

1kg (2.2lb) lamb shoulder, cubed

200g (7oz) spinach

3 tablespoons coriander (cilantro) chopped

2 onions, finely chopped

2 cloves of garlic, finely chopped

2.5cm (1inch) chunk of ginger, grated (shredded)

2 chillies, finely chopped

1 teaspoon paprika

1 teaspoon turmeric

1 teaspoon ground coriander (cilantro)

2 tablespoons plain Greek yogurt

3 tablespoons coconut oil

250mls lamb or beef stock (broth)

Sea salt, freshly ground black pepper

SERVES 4-6

Method

Place the ginger, chillies, coriander, garlic, spices and yogurt into a blender and process until smooth. Cover the meat with the marinade and chill for at least an hour or overnight if you can. Heat the coconut oil in a pan, add the onion and cook for 5 minutes. Add the marinated meat and cook for 2 minutes. Pour in the stock (broth) and simmer for 1 hour, stirring occasionally and adding extra stock or water if required. Stir in the spinach and cook for another 10 minutes.

Pork Koftas & Roast Pepper Salad

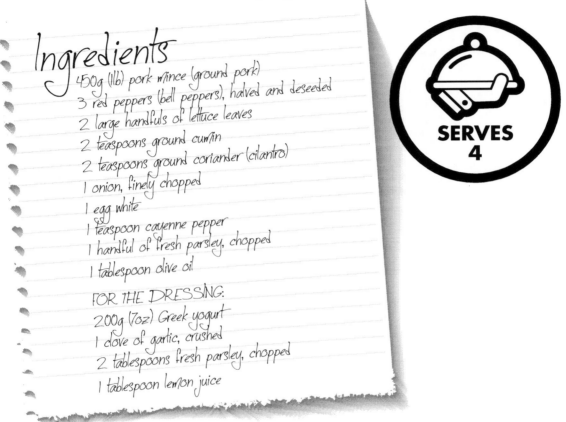

Ingredients

450g (1lb) pork mince (ground pork)

3 red peppers (bell peppers), halved and deseeded

2 large handfuls of lettuce leaves

2 teaspoons ground cumin

2 teaspoons ground coriander (cilantro)

1 onion, finely chopped

1 egg white

1 teaspoon cayenne pepper

1 handful of fresh parsley, chopped

1 tablespoon olive oil

FOR THE DRESSING:

200g (7oz) Greek yogurt

1 clove of garlic, crushed

2 tablespoons fresh parsley, chopped

1 tablespoon lemon juice

SERVES 4

Method

Place the peppers (bell peppers) under a hot grill (broiler) and cook until the skin is charred. Place the peppers into a bag for 3 minutes until the skin loosens them peel it off. Chop the peppers and set aside. Heat the olive oil in a pan, add the onion and cook until softened. Stir in the spices and cook for 2 minutes. In a bowl, combine the onions, pork, egg white and parsley. Make the mixture into 8 sausage shapes and slide them onto skewers. Place them under a hot grill (broiler) and cook for about 8 minutes, turning occasionally until completely cooked. Combine the dressing ingredients into a bowl. Serve the lettuce leaves and chopped peppers onto plates. Add the koftas on top and serve with a spoonful of dressing.

Chicken & Mushroom Cream Sauce

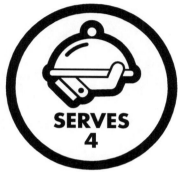

SERVES 4

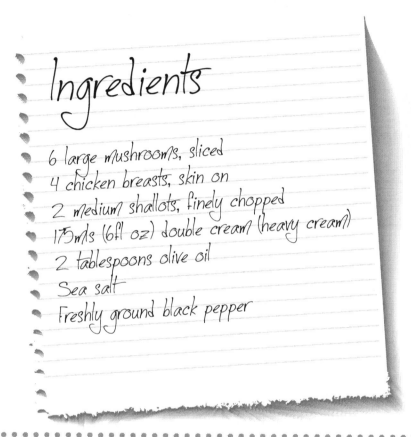

Ingredients

- 6 large mushrooms, sliced
- 4 chicken breasts, skin on
- 2 medium shallots, finely chopped
- 175mls (6fl oz) double cream (heavy cream)
- 2 tablespoons olive oil
- Sea salt
- Freshly ground black pepper

Method

Heat the olive oil in a frying pan. Add the chicken breasts and cook them for around 7 minutes on either side or until cooked through as the thickness can vary. Transfer the chicken to a plate and cover it with foil to keep it warm. Add the mushrooms and the shallots to the pan and cook until they have softened. Pour in the cream and season with salt and pepper. Stir until warmed through. Serve the chicken breasts with the sauce.

Chilli Garlic Cod

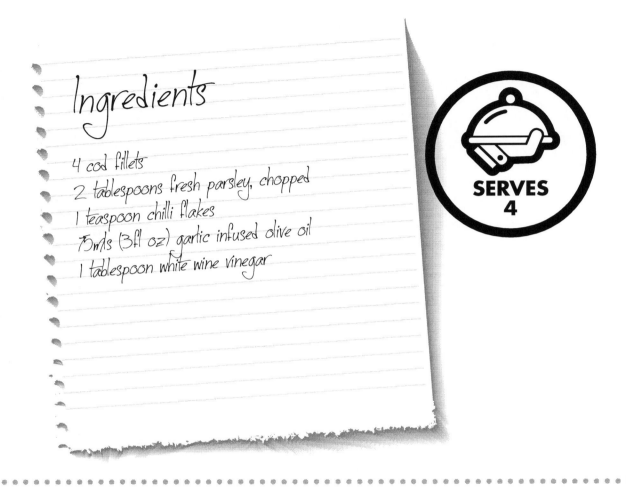

Ingredients

4 cod fillets
2 tablespoons fresh parsley, chopped
1 teaspoon chilli flakes
75mls (3fl oz) garlic infused olive oil
1 tablespoon white wine vinegar

SERVES 4

Method

Heat a tablespoon of olive oil in a frying pan, add the fish and cook until cooked through, turning once halfway through. Remove and keep warm. Place the olive oil, chilli, parsley and vinegar in the frying pan and warm it through. Serve the fish and pour the oil over.

Fillet Steak With Garlic & Chive Butter

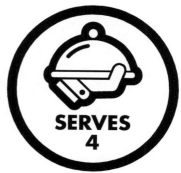

SERVES 4

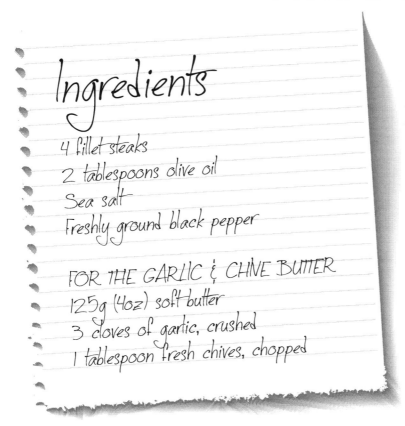

Ingredients

4 fillet steaks
2 tablespoons olive oil
Sea salt
Freshly ground black pepper

FOR THE GARLIC & CHIVE BUTTER
125g (4oz) soft butter
3 cloves of garlic, crushed
1 tablespoon fresh chives, chopped

Method

Place the butter in a bowl with the garlic and chives and combine until smooth. Chill the butter in the fridge for 20 minutes. Sprinkle the steaks with salt and pepper. Heat the olive oil in a frying pan and add the steaks. Cook them to your liking. As a guide 2½ minutes each side for rare, 3 ½ minutes each side for medium rare and 4½ minutes each side for medium. Serve the steaks with a large spoonful of garlic butter on top. Allow them to rest for 5 minutes before eating.

Lamb & Gorgonzola Burgers

SERVES 4

Ingredients

450g (1lb) minced (ground) lamb

8 small slices Gorgonzola cheese

1 onion, finely chopped

1 egg, beaten

1 clove garlic, crushed

2 tablespoons chives, finely chopped

2 tablespoons olive oil

8 lettuce leaves

Sea salt

Freshly ground black pepper

Method

Place the lamb, egg, onion, garlic and chives in a bowl and combine the ingredients. Season with salt and pepper. Shape the mixture into 8 small round patties. Heat the olive oil in a frying pan, add the burgers and cook for 5-6 minutes on each side. Add a slice of cheese to each burger and let it melt. Serve the cheeseburgers in a lettuce leaf wrap. You can also add sliced avocado and tomato if you wish.

Feta, Egg & Green Pepper Salad

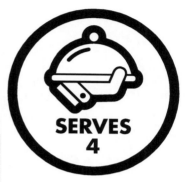

SERVES 4

Ingredients

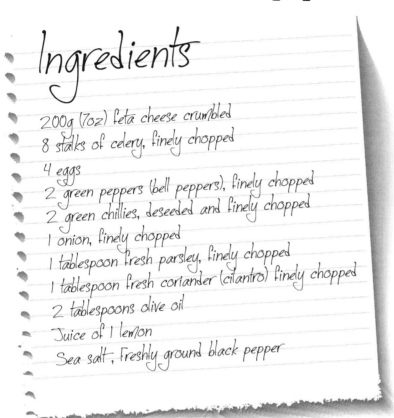

200g (7oz) feta cheese crumbled

8 stalks of celery, finely chopped

4 eggs

2 green peppers (bell peppers), finely chopped

2 green chillies, deseeded and finely chopped

1 onion, finely chopped

1 tablespoon fresh parsley, finely chopped

1 tablespoon fresh coriander (cilantro) finely chopped

2 tablespoons olive oil

Juice of 1 lemon

Sea salt, freshly ground black pepper

Method

Place the green peppers, celery, onion, parsley, coriander (cilantro) chilli, olive oil and lemon juice in a bowl. Season with salt and pepper and mix well. Allow the vegetables to marinate for 30 minutes. When ready to serve, bring a pan of water to the boil, add the eggs and cook for 5 minutes then remove them from the heat and run them under cold water. Remove the egg shells. Serve the marinated salad onto plates, sprinkle the feta cheese over and add an egg cut in half onto the salad. Serve and eat immediately.

Baked Tarragon Chicken

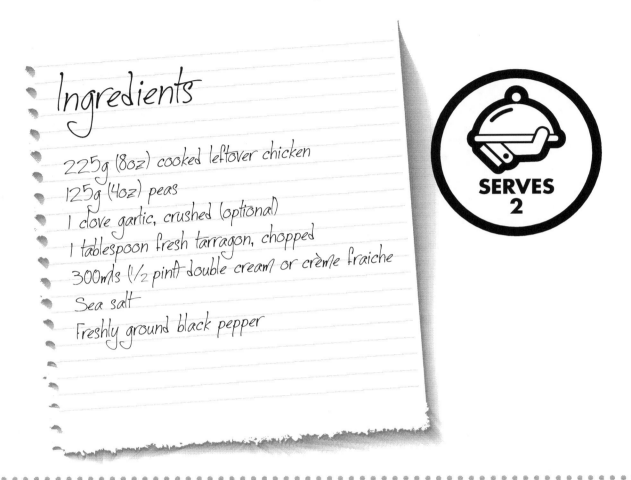

Ingredients

225g (8oz) cooked leftover chicken
125g (4oz) peas
1 clove garlic, crushed (optional)
1 tablespoon fresh tarragon, chopped
300mls (½ pint) double cream or crème fraiche
Sea salt
Freshly ground black pepper

SERVES
2

Method

Scatter the chicken and peas in an ovenproof dish. Add the garlic (if using) and tarragon. Pour over the cream and season with salt and pepper. Transfer it to the oven and bake for 20 minutes, checking it is hot throughout. Serve with a salad or steamed mixed vegetables.

Beef Satay Skewers

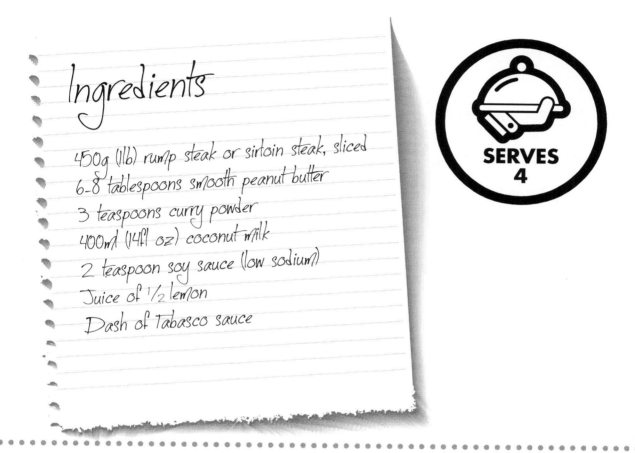

Ingredients

450g (1lb) rump steak or sirloin steak, sliced
6-8 tablespoons smooth peanut butter
3 teaspoons curry powder
400ml (14fl oz) coconut milk
2 teaspoon soy sauce (low sodium)
Juice of 1/2 lemon
Dash of Tabasco sauce

SERVES 4

Method

In a bowl, combine the peanut butter and coconut milk. Stir in the curry powder, Tabasco and soy sauce. Thoroughly coat the beef pieces in the peanut mixture. Thread the beef onto skewers, and set aside the remaining satay sauce. Place the beef skewers under a hot grill (broiler) and cook for 4-5 minutes on each side, making sure they are thoroughly cooked. Pour the remaining satay sauce into a small saucepan add lemon juice and bring to the boil. Serve the chicken skewers and pour the remaining satay sauce on top.

Roast Red Pepper Chicken

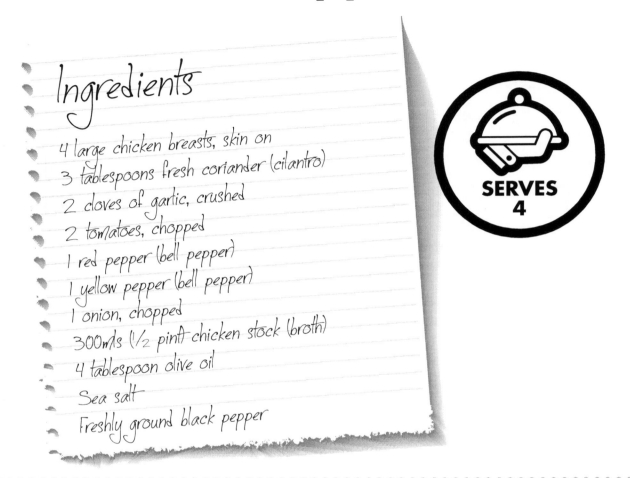

Ingredients

4 large chicken breasts, skin on
3 tablespoons fresh coriander (cilantro)
2 cloves of garlic, crushed
2 tomatoes, chopped
1 red pepper (bell pepper)
1 yellow pepper (bell pepper)
1 onion, chopped
300mls (1/2 pint) chicken stock (broth)
4 tablespoon olive oil
Sea salt
Freshly ground black pepper

SERVES 4

Method

Heat the olive oil in a frying pan, add the chicken and brown it for 5 minutes. Add the garlic and onions and cook for 5 minutes. Add the peppers (bell peppers), tomatoes and chicken stock (broth) bring it to the boil, reduce the heat and simmer for 15 minutes. Stir in the fresh coriander (cilantro) and season with salt and pepper. Serve with avocado and salad.

Salmon & Watercress Cream

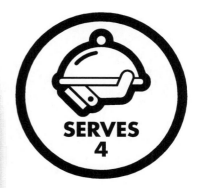

SERVES
4

Ingredients

4 salmon fillets
25g (1oz) butter
1 handful of watercress, finely chopped
1 clove garlic, crushed
300mls (10fl oz) crème fraiche
100mls (3½ fl oz) vegetable stock (broth)
1 tablespoon olive oil
Sea salt, freshly ground black pepper

Method

Heat the olive oil in a frying pan, add the salmon fillets and cook for around 9 minutes until the fish is thoroughly cooked, turning once during cooking. Remove the fish from the pan, cover and keep warm. Place the butter and garlic in the pan and cook for around a minute. Pour in the stock (broth) and bring it to the boil then reduce the heat. Stir in the crème fraiche to the pan and cook for 3 minutes. Add the watercress and cook until it softens. Season with salt and pepper. Serve the salmon and pour over the watercress cream. Enjoy.

Roast Garlic & Rosemary Lamb

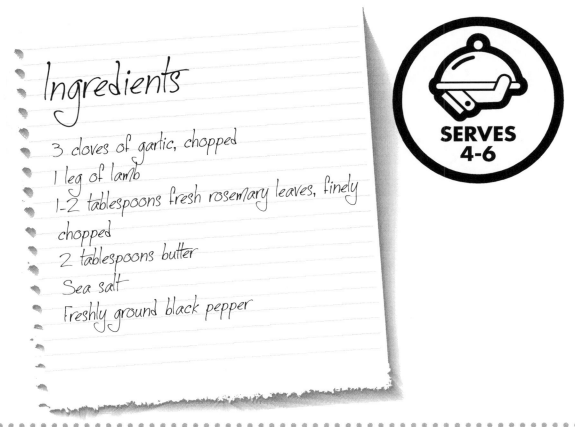

SERVES 4-6

Ingredients

3 cloves of garlic, chopped

1 leg of lamb

1-2 tablespoons fresh rosemary leaves, finely chopped

2 tablespoons butter

Sea salt

Freshly ground black pepper

Method

Place the garlic and rosemary in a pestle in mortar and grind to a smooth paste. Mix it with the butter until well combined. Make several incisions in the lamb and press the herby butter into the cuts and spread the rest over the lamb. Season the lamb with salt and pepper. Place the lamb in a roasting tin and cook until the lamb is done to your liking. It will take around 20 minutes for each 450g (1lb) of meat. Serve with vegetables or salad.

Cajun Swordfish

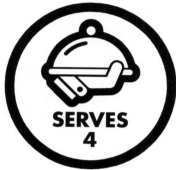

SERVES 4

Ingredients

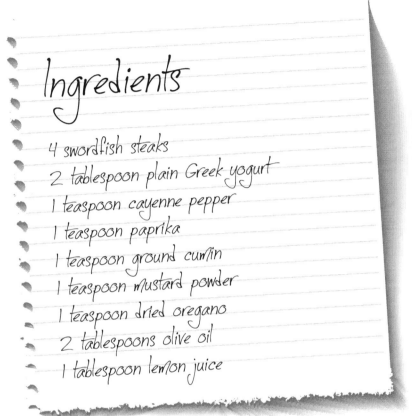

4 swordfish steaks
2 tablespoon plain Greek yogurt
1 teaspoon cayenne pepper
1 teaspoon paprika
1 teaspoon ground cumin
1 teaspoon mustard powder
1 teaspoon dried oregano
2 tablespoons olive oil
1 tablespoon lemon juice

Method

Mix the spices together in a bowl and set aside. Mix the yogurt and lemon juice in a bowl and coat the fish in the yogurt mixture. Pat the spices into the coated fish making sure it's well covered. Heat the olive oil in a frying pan or griddle pan and add the fish. Cook for around 10 minutes, turning once half-way through until the fish is completely cooked. Serve and enjoy.

Chicken & Cashew Korma

Ingredients

4 skinless chicken breasts, chopped
3 tablespoons Greek yogurt
1 teaspoon ground ginger
1 garlic clove, crushed
1/2 teaspoon garam masala

FOR THE SAUCE:
50g (2oz) cashew nuts
2 garlic cloves, crushed
1 onion, finely chopped
1 tablespoon coconut oil
200mls (7fl oz) chicken stock (broth)
150g (6oz) Greek yogurt
1 large handful of spinach leaves
2 tablespoons coriander (cilantro) leaves, chopped

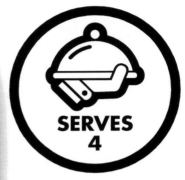

SERVES 4

Method

Combine the chicken, yogurt, garam masala, ginger and garlic in a bowl and marinate for 1 hour. Place the onion and garlic into a food processor and blitz until a smooth paste. Heat the coconut oil in a pan, add the chicken and marinade and brown the chicken. Stir the onion and garlic mixture into the pan and the stock (broth). Bring to the boil, reduce the heat and simmer for 15 minutes. Place the cashews and yogurt into a food processor and blitz until smooth. Add the yogurt mixture, spinach and coriander (cilantro) to the pan and cook until the spinach has wilted. Serve and enjoy.

Mushroom & Tarragon Pork

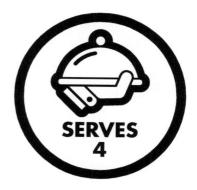

SERVES
4

Ingredients

- 450g (1lb) pork steaks
- 300g (11oz) mushrooms
- 1 tablespoons fresh tarragon leaves, chopped
- 300mls (1/2 pint) crème fraiche
- 4 tablespoons olive oil
- Juice of 1/2 lemon
- Sea salt
- Freshly ground black pepper

Method

Heat the olive oil in a pan, add the pork and brown them for 3 minutes. Remove and set aside. Place the mushrooms in the frying pan and cook for 5 minutes until soft. Return the pork to the pan and add in the crème fraiche and tarragon. Squeeze in the lemon juice and season with salt and pepper. Simmer for 5 minutes. Serve with steamed vegetables or salad.

Paprika King Prawns & Chilli Herb Dressing

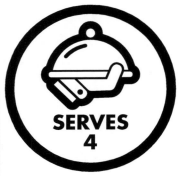

SERVES 4

Ingredients

24 large peeled raw king prawns (shrimps)

1 tablespoon coconut oil or olive oil

FOR THE DRESSING:

2 cloves of garlic

2 tablespoons capers

1 small handful of coriander (cilantro) leaves, chopped

1 small handful of fresh parsley, chopped

3 tablespoons white wine vinegar

6 tablespoons olive oil

1 bag of fresh green salad leaves

Method

For the dressing, place the oil, garlic, capers, herbs and vinegar into a bowl and stir. Place the prawns in a separate bowl and pour over **half** of the dressing. Allow the prawns to marinate for as long as you can, preferably overnight. Cover the remaining dressing and store in the fridge until ready to use. Heat a tablespoon of olive oil or coconut oil into a frying pan, add the prawns and cook for around 3 minutes until they turn pink and are completely cooked. Serve the salad onto plates, add the cooked prawns and drizzle the remaining dressing.

Thai Pork Parcels

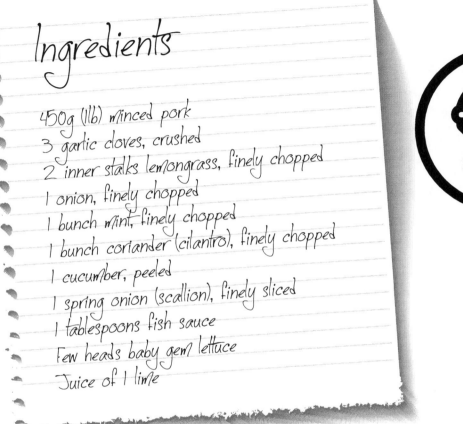

Ingredients

450g (1lb) minced pork
3 garlic cloves, crushed
2 inner stalks lemongrass, finely chopped
1 onion, finely chopped
1 bunch mint, finely chopped
1 bunch coriander (cilantro), finely chopped
1 cucumber, peeled
1 spring onion (scallion), finely sliced
1 tablespoons fish sauce
Few heads baby gem lettuce
Juice of 1 lime

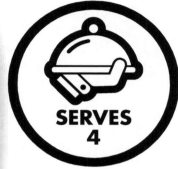

SERVES
4

Method

Place the pork, garlic, lemongrass, onion and fish sauce into a bowl and combine them well. Shape the mixture into patties and place them on a lightly greased baking tray. Transfer them to the oven and bake at 200C/400F for 15–20 minutes. Meanwhile, you can make little salad boats to serve them in. Grate (shred) a cucumber without the skin and mix with the sliced spring onion (scallion). Serve the pork parcels into the lettuce leaves and add the cucumber and spring onion. Sprinkle with coriander (cilantro) and mint and a squeeze of lime juice.

Lemon Butter Chicken

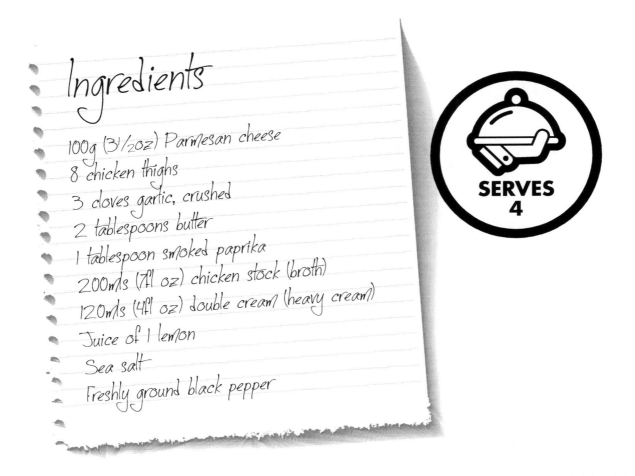

Ingredients

100g (3½oz) Parmesan cheese

8 chicken thighs

3 cloves garlic, crushed

2 tablespoons butter

1 tablespoon smoked paprika

200mls (7fl oz) chicken stock (broth)

120mls (4fl oz) double cream (heavy cream)

Juice of 1 lemon

Sea salt

Freshly ground black pepper

SERVES 4

Method

Sprinkle the chicken with paprika, salt and pepper. Heat the butter in a frying pan, add the chicken and brown it on both sides for around 2-3 minutes. Remove the chicken and set it aside. Add the garlic to the pan and cook it for 2 minutes. Pour in the chicken stock (broth), parmesan, cream and lemon juice. Bring it to the boil, reduce the heat and simmer for 2 minutes. Return the chicken to the pan. Simmer gently for around 20 minutes or until the chicken is completely cooked. Serve with a green salad onto a bed of fresh spinach.

Coconut Crumb Prawns

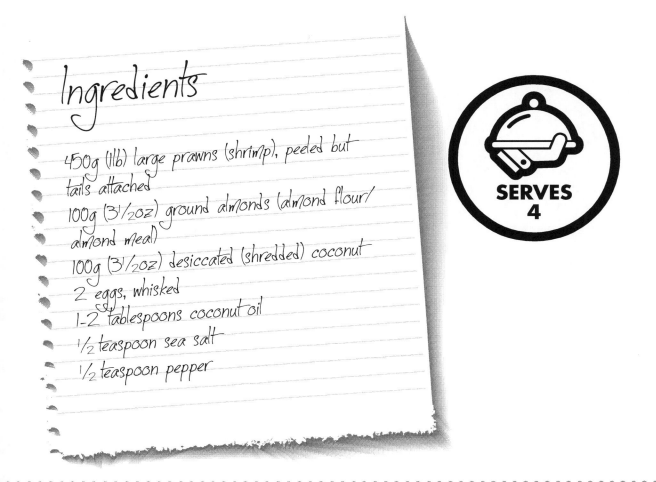

Ingredients

450g (1lb) large prawns (shrimp), peeled but tails attached

100g (3½oz) ground almonds (almond flour/ almond meal)

100g (3½oz) desiccated (shredded) coconut

2 eggs, whisked

1-2 tablespoons coconut oil

½ teaspoon sea salt

½ teaspoon pepper

SERVES 4

Method

Place the ground almonds, salt and pepper into a bowl, in another bowl place the beaten egg and in another place the desiccated (shredded) coconut. Dip the prawns (shrimp) in the ground almonds (almond flour/ almond meal) then dip them in the eggs and finally dredge it in the coconut making sure you get plenty of coconut onto each one for crispiness. Continue for each of the prawns and set them onto a plate. Place enough oil in a large pan, enough to completely cover the bottom. Add a few prawns at a time and cook for around 2-3 minutes on each side. Serve with mayonnaise.

Turkey Curry

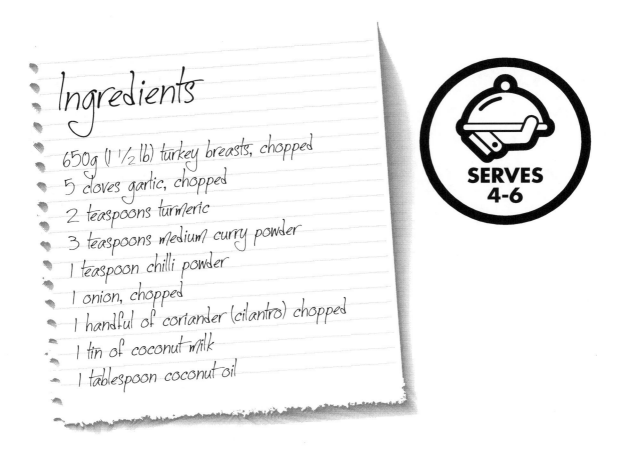

Ingredients

- 650g (1 ½ lb) turkey breasts, chopped
- 5 cloves garlic, chopped
- 2 teaspoons turmeric
- 3 teaspoons medium curry powder
- 1 teaspoon chilli powder
- 1 onion, chopped
- 1 handful of coriander (cilantro) chopped
- 1 tin of coconut milk
- 1 tablespoon coconut oil

SERVES 4-6

Method

Heat the coconut oil in a saucepan, add the onion and cook it for 5 minutes. Stir in the garlic and the turkey and cook it for 7-8 minutes. Add the spices and stir well into the other ingredients. Pour in the coconut milk and coriander (cilantro). Bring it to the boil, reduce the heat and simmer for around 10 minutes. Serve with cauliflower rice (see recipe).

Baked Chicory

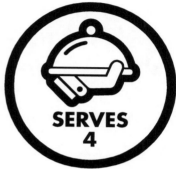

SERVES
4

Ingredients

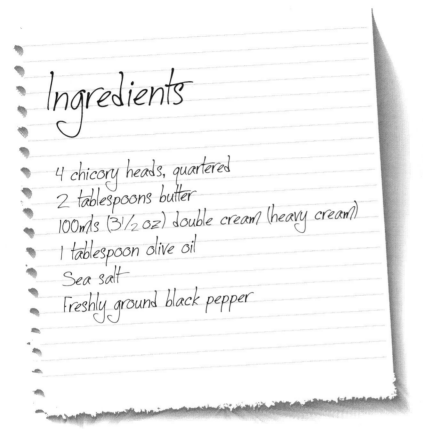

4 chicory heads, quartered
2 tablespoons butter
100mls (3½ oz) double cream (heavy cream)
1 tablespoon olive oil
Sea salt
Freshly ground black pepper

Method

Grease a casserole dish with the olive oil and place the chicory in the dish. Flake the butter over the chicory and season with a little salt and pepper. Cover the dish with foil and transfer it to the oven. Bake at 190C/375F for 45 minutes, basting the chicory occasionally. Remove it from the oven and add the cream to the chicory. Place it under a hot grill (broiler) until golden. Serve as a carbohydrate alternative to potatoes, rice and pasta.

Fried 'Rice'

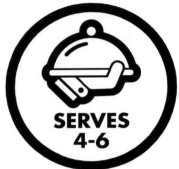

SERVES 4-6

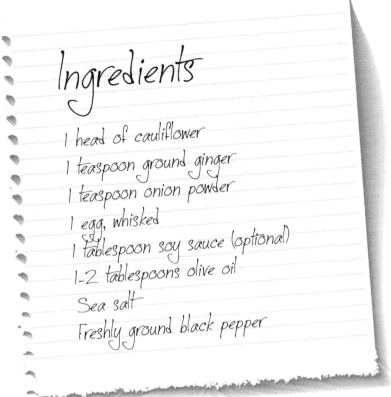

Ingredients

1 head of cauliflower
1 teaspoon ground ginger
1 teaspoon onion powder
1 egg, whisked
1 tablespoon soy sauce (optional)
1-2 tablespoons olive oil
Sea salt
Freshly ground black pepper

Method

Place the cauliflower into a food processor and chop until fine, similar to rice. Heat the oil in a frying pan. Stir in the ginger, onion powder and the cauliflower. Cook for around 6 minutes or until softened. Towards the end of cooking, move the cauliflower to one side of the pan, making a space for the egg. Pour the egg into the space and stir it briskly with a fork, breaking it up. Once it's cooked stir it throughout the rice along with the soy sauce (optional). Season with salt and pepper and serve.

Curried Cauliflower Rice

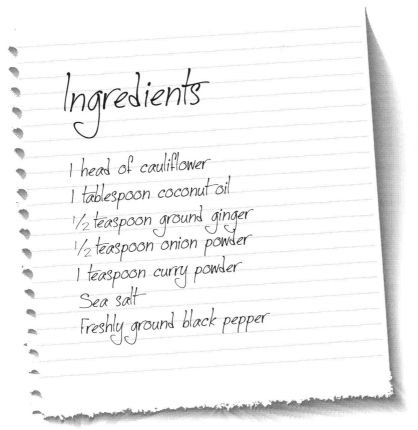

Ingredients

1 head of cauliflower
1 tablespoon coconut oil
½ teaspoon ground ginger
½ teaspoon onion powder
1 teaspoon curry powder
Sea salt
Freshly ground black pepper

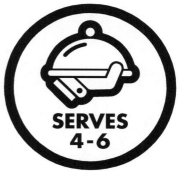

SERVES 4-6

Method

Place the cauliflower into a food processor and chop until fine, similar to rice. Heat the coconut oil in a frying pan. Stir in the ginger, curry powder, onion powder and the cauliflower. Cook for around 6 minutes or until softened. Serve as an alternative to rice. You can replace the ginger and curry powder with a little onion powder if you wish to have it plain but still full of flavour.

DESSERTS, TREATS & SNACKS

Chocolate Ice Cream

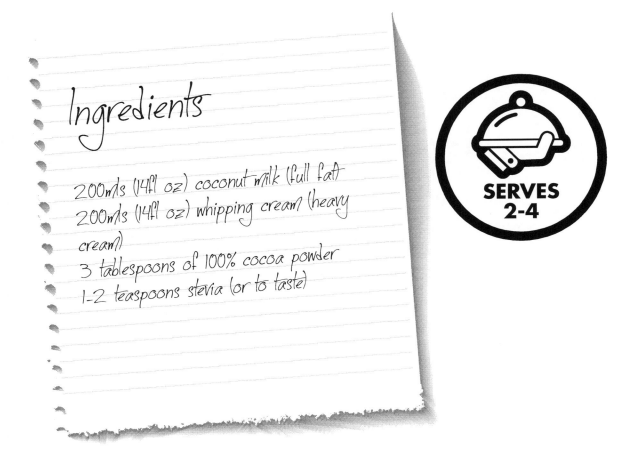

Ingredients

200mls (14fl oz) coconut milk (full fat)
200mls (14fl oz) whipping cream (heavy cream)
3 tablespoons of 100% cocoa powder
1-2 teaspoons stevia (or to taste)

SERVES
2-4

Method

In a bowl, whip the cream until thick. Stir in the coconut milk, cocoa powder and stevia and mix really well. Once the mixture has been whisked you can transfer it to a freezer or an ice cream maker and process it for the required time depending on your machine. Freeze or eat straight away.

Lemon Cheesecake

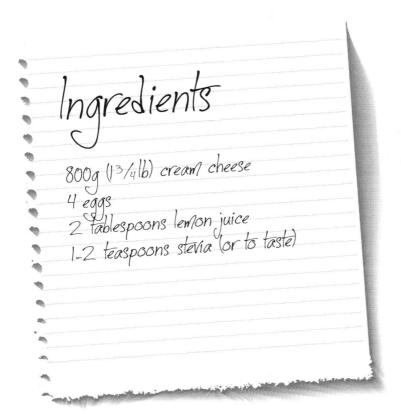

Ingredients

800g (1¾lb) cream cheese
4 eggs
2 tablespoons lemon juice
1-2 teaspoons stevia (or to taste)

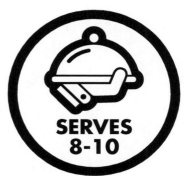

SERVES
8-10

Method

Place all of the ingredients into a bowl and combine them. Transfer the mixture to a pie dish and bake at 170C/325F for one hour. Remove the cheesecake and allow it to cool. Serve chilled.

Coconut Truffles

Ingredients

100g (3½ oz) cream cheese
3 tablespoons desiccated (shredded) coconut
2 tablespoons coconut oil
3 tablespoons creamed coconut
Pinch of salt
Juice of a lemon
1 teaspoons stevia (or to taste)

For the coating: ¼ cup desiccated (shredded) coconut

SERVES 4

Method

Blend together the coconut oil and the cream cheese. Add the in creamed coconut, stevia, lemon juice and a pinch of salt. Mix in the 3 tablespoons of desiccated (shredded) coconut. Chill in the fridge until the mixture becomes firm. Roll the mixture into balls and roll it in the coconut. Store in the fridge until ready to eat.

Peanut & Chocolate Brittle

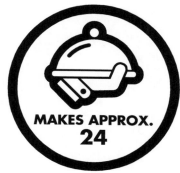

MAKES APPROX.
24

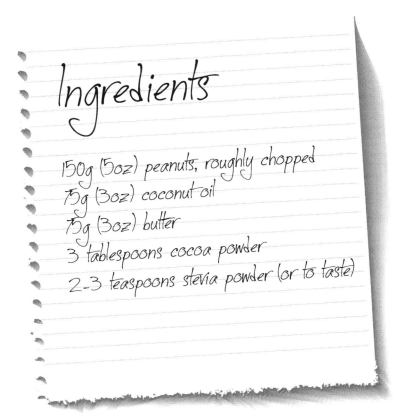

Ingredients

150g (5oz) peanuts, roughly chopped

75g (3oz) coconut oil

75g (3oz) butter

3 tablespoons cocoa powder

2-3 teaspoons stevia powder (or to taste)

Method

Place the coconut oil and butter in a saucepan. Mix in the stevia and cocoa powder and stir until mixed well. Spread half of the peanuts nuts in the bottom of a small loaf tin or dish. Cover the peanuts with HALF of the chocolate mixture. Sprinkle on top the remaining peanuts and pour on the remaining chocolate. Place it in the fridge and chill until the chocolate has hardened. Cut it into approximately 24 rough chunks and serve. Keep refrigerated until ready to eat.

Orange & Ginger Mousse

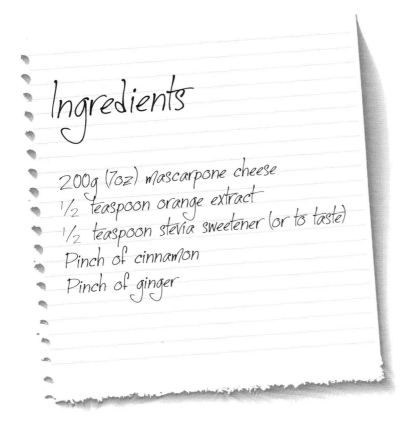

Ingredients

200g (7oz) mascarpone cheese
½ teaspoon orange extract
½ teaspoon stevia sweetener (or to taste)
Pinch of cinnamon
Pinch of ginger

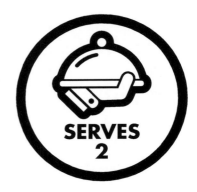

SERVES
2

Method

Place the mascarpone into a blender along with the stevia, orange extract and spices. Process until smooth. Transfer to serving bowls and chill before serving.

Pecan Truffles

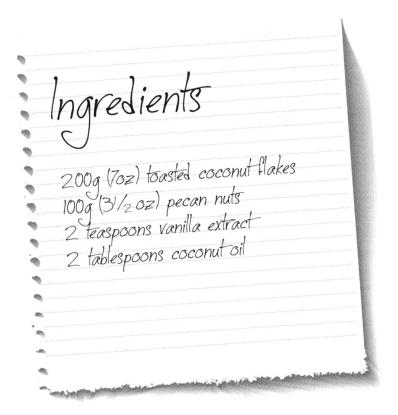

Ingredients

200g (7oz) toasted coconut flakes
100g (3½ oz) pecan nuts
2 teaspoons vanilla extract
2 tablespoons coconut oil

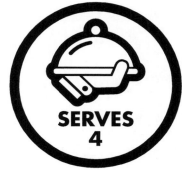

SERVES 4

Method

Place all of the ingredients into a blender and process until smooth and creamy. Add a little extra coconut oil if required. Divide the mixture into bite-size pieces and roll it into balls. Place the balls into small paper cake cases. Chill before serving.

Coffee Creams

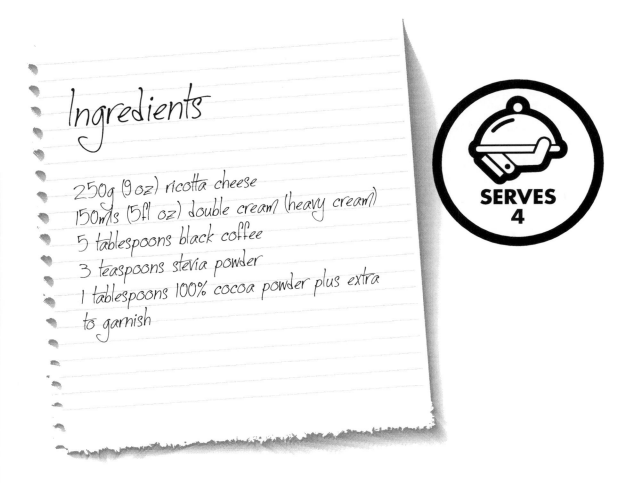

Ingredients

250g (9 oz) ricotta cheese
150mls (5fl oz) double cream (heavy cream)
5 tablespoons black coffee
3 teaspoons stevia powder
1 tablespoons 100% cocoa powder plus extra
to garnish

SERVES 4

Method

Mix together the coffee and stevia and stir it well. Place the ricotta into a bowl and beat it to soften it then pour in the coffee mixture and combine it. Whisk the double cream (heavy cream) until it forms soft peaks. Fold the whisked cream into the ricotta mixture and stir in the cocoa powder. Combine the mixture well. Spoon it into dessert glasses or decorative bowls. Sprinkle with a little cocoa powder and chill before serving.

Chocolate Shake

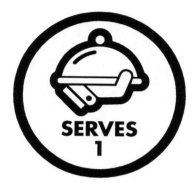

SERVES
1

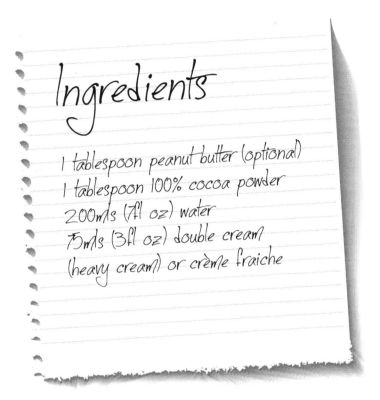

Ingredients

1 tablespoon peanut butter (optional)
1 tablespoon 100% cocoa powder
200mls (7fl oz) water
75mls (3fl oz) double cream
(heavy cream) or crème fraiche

Method

Place all of the ingredients into a blender and process until smooth. Serve with a few ice cubes in a tall glass. You can leave out the peanut butter and add in a mint leaf or two for a delicious minty chocolate shake.

Chocolate Coated Coconut Snack Bars

Ingredients

FOR THE SNACK BARS
100g (3½ oz) desiccated (shredded) coconut
½-1 teaspoon stevia sweetener
1 tablespoon coconut oil
1 teaspoon vanilla extract
60mls (2fl oz) coconut cream

FOR THE TOPPING
½-1 teaspoons stevia powder
4 tablespoons coconut oil
2 tablespoons 100% cocoa powder

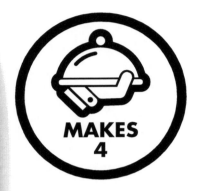

MAKES
4

Method

Place all of the ingredients for the snack bars into a food processer and process until smooth. Taste test the sweetness and add a little extra sweetener if you wish. Line a small rectangular baking tin or baking sheet with parchment paper. Press the coconut mixture into a rectangular shape and cut the mixture into bars of around 1 inch thick (or to your liking). Transfer the coconut bars to the fridge and chill until completely solid. When ready for the topping, place the coconut oil, cocoa powder and stevia into a saucepan on a low heat for 2-3 minutes. Allow the chocolate mixture to cool but remain liquid. Dip the coconut bars in the chocolate and coat them well. Place the bars on a plate and place them in the fridge to harden. Enjoy.

Almond Butter Cups

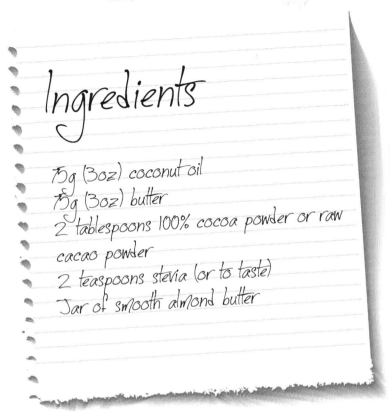

Ingredients

75g (3oz) coconut oil
75g (3oz) butter
2 tablespoons 100% cocoa powder or raw cacao powder
2 teaspoons stevia (or to taste)
Jar of smooth almond butter

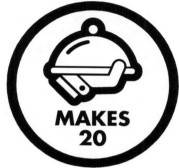

MAKES
20

Method

Place the butter, coconut oil, cocoa powder and stevia powder into a saucepan and gently warm it until the chocolate mixture is smooth. Lay out some very small paper cake cases to hold bite-size amounts. Spoon half the liquid chocolate mixture into the bottom of the paper cases and fill them only ½ way. Let them cool slightly. Add a teaspoon of almond butter to each of the cases. Sometimes you need to warm the chocolate a little more if it starts to solidify. Spoon the remainder of the chocolate into the cases and cover the almond butter. Chill in the fridge for 1-2 hours before serving.

CONDIMENTS

Red Cabbage & Walnut Coleslaw

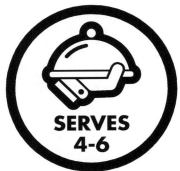

SERVES 4-6

Ingredients

½ red cabbage, finely grated (shredded)

3 stalks of celery, finely chopped

2 tablespoons chopped walnuts

4 tablespoons mayonnaise (sugar-free)

Sea salt

Freshly ground black pepper

Method

Place the cabbage, celery, walnuts and mayonnaise into a bowl and combine the ingredients well. Add extra mayonnaise to coat the vegetables thoroughly if you need to. Season with salt and pepper. Chill before serving.

Herb Cheese

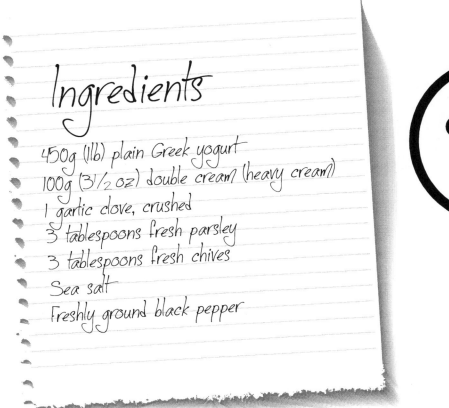

Ingredients

450g (1lb) plain Greek yogurt
100g (3½ oz) double cream (heavy cream)
1 garlic clove, crushed
3 tablespoons fresh parsley
3 tablespoons fresh chives
Sea salt
Freshly ground black pepper

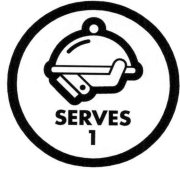

SERVES 1

Method

Place all of the ingredients into a bowl and mix well. Using a piece of muslin line a separate bowl and add the yogurt and cream mixture into the muslin. Draw the edges of the muslin together to make a bag to drain the excess moisture off the mixture. Tie a band around the end of the bag and suspend the bag over a bowl overnight. In the morning, scoop the cheese into a bowl. Stir in the garlic, herbs, salt and pepper. Cover it and chill before serving. Serve scooped onto chopped vegetables.

Tzatziki

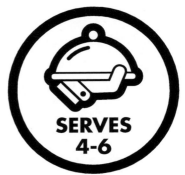

SERVES 4-6

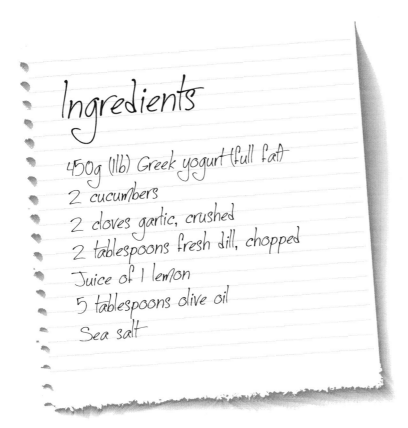

Ingredients

450g (1lb) Greek yogurt (full fat)

2 cucumbers

2 cloves garlic, crushed

2 tablespoons fresh dill, chopped

Juice of 1 lemon

5 tablespoons olive oil

Sea salt

Method

Grate (shred) the cucumber into a colander and sprinkle with salt. Squeeze out the excess moisture and let it drain for 30 minutes or more. Place the yogurt into a bowl and add the cucumber, garlic, olive oil, lemon juice and dill. Mix well. Transfer the tzatziki to a serving dish and chill well before serving.

Almond & Coriander (Cilantro) Pesto

Ingredients

50g (2oz) blanched almonds
25g (1oz) pine nuts
2 tablespoons Parmesan, grated
2 cloves garlic, crushed
1 large handful of fresh coriander (cilantro)
175mls (6fl oz) olive oil
Sea salt
Freshly ground black pepper

Method

In a pan, dry fry the pine nuts and almonds until golden. Place all of the ingredients into a food processor and blitz until it becomes smooth.

Pistachio & Basil Pesto

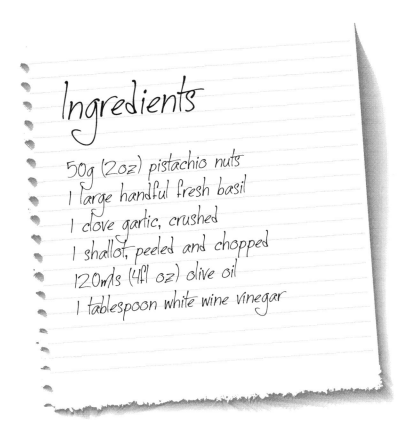

Ingredients

50g (2oz) pistachio nuts
1 large handful fresh basil
1 clove garlic, crushed
1 shallot, peeled and chopped
120mls (4fl oz) olive oil
1 tablespoon white wine vinegar

Method

Place all of the ingredients into a food processor and blitz until smooth.

Lemon & Chilli Mayonnaise

Ingredients

2 teaspoons lemon juice
2 egg yolks
300mls (10fl oz) olive oil
½-1 teaspoon chilli flakes (or to taste)
Sea salt
Freshly ground black pepper

Method

Place the egg yolks and lemon juice into a blender and process until smooth and frothy. Slowly add in the olive oil a little at a time and blend until it's shiny and thick. Stir in the chilli flakes and season with salt and pepper.

16696891R00069

Printed in Great Britain
by Amazon